PREVENTING
LOW BACK PAIN

PREVENTING LOW BACK PAIN

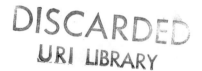
Paul D. Hooper, DC

Chair

Department of Principles and Practice

Los Angeles College of Chiropractic

Whittier, California

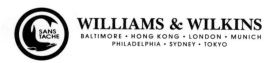
WILLIAMS & WILKINS
BALTIMORE · HONG KONG · LONDON · MUNICH
PHILADELPHIA · SYDNEY · TOKYO

Editor: Jonathan W. Pine, Jr.
Managing Editor: Marjorie Kidd Keating
Copy Editor: Janet M. Krejci
Designer: Dan Pfisterer
Illustration Planner: Lorraine Wrzosek
Production Coordinator: Anne Stewart Seitz
Cover Designers: Dan Pfisterer/Mike Kotarba

Printed in the United States of America

Library of Congress Cataloging in Publication Data

Hooper, Paul D.
   Preventing low back pain / Paul D. Hooper.
     p. cm.
   Includes index.
   ISBN 0–683–04873–2
   1. Backache—Prevention.   2. Backache—Chiropractic treatment.
I. Title.
   [DNLM: 1. Backache—prevention & control.   WE 755 H787p]
RZ265.S64H66   1992
617.5' 64—dc20
DNLM/DLC
for Library of Congress   91–44670
                                           CIP

                     92 93 94 95 96
      1 2 3 4 5 6 7 8 9 10

Preface

Back pain is one of the most common and costly problems encountered by the health care system. Countless texts and articles have been written on the topic. Seminars and symposia abound. Billions of dollars are spent annually on the various aspects of back pain.

Unlike numerous other health problems, back pain is a problem for many of the clinicians treating back pain patients. My own interest in the topic stems, in part, from my own back problems. Likewise, my interest in methods of prevention also stems from my own experience.

During the course of writing *Preventing Low Back Pain*, I was confronted with a most difficult and challenging experience. As described in the last part of the text, a close friend of mine suffered a serious back injury. I saw his physical condition worsen and I also saw his state of mind deteriorate. His case was a textbook example of all the things that can go wrong with the system. Fortunately, during the time since completion of the manuscript for this text, my friend has recovered. To a great extent, I attribute his recovery to a change in his attitude rather than any one thing that was done for him clinically. This change was initiated during a visit with Dr. Scott Haldeman in which my friend was "challenged" to get better. His recovery since that time has been nothing short of remarkable.

I am firmly convinced that the solution to the back pain problem will not be found in better diagnostic or treatment methods. Everybody involved must modify their approach. Clinicians must resist the temptation to disable the patient by magnifying the seriousness of the condition. Today's clinicians must encourage patients to become involved in their own recovery and must find ways of facilitating patients' activity. Greater emphasis must be placed on education of the injured individual as a treatment tool. Employers must change their attitudes toward workers with back injury. Every attempt should be made to facilitate an early return to work and to provide a cooperative rather than adversarial environment. In addition, employers should promote good health practices in the work place. Providers must encourage injury prevention programs and should provide preferential status to patients in active rehabilitation programs. Lastly, patients must accept responsibility for their own recovery.

My thanks to Debbie, Alison, and Benjie for their patience during the writing of this text. Thanks also to Steve Foreman for providing me with the mechanism to express my ideas and thoughts.

Contents

1

Statistics Relating to Back Pain

Each text written on the subject of back pain includes an introductory chapter that deals with the high incidence and the staggering costs of the problem. It is abundantly clear from the large amount of accumulated data that back pain is one of the most frequent and costly health problems that face modern man. The purpose of this chapter is not simply to repeat the same statistics that appear elsewhere. Rather, we will look at the statistics in an effort to gain a better understanding of the problem.

Back pain is not a new problem. Since ancient times man has been afflicted with back problems. Many old medical textbooks, some dating back to the days of Hippocrates, contain illustrations and descriptions of a diversity of treatment methods aimed at lumbago, rheumatism, and sciatica. In his text on Autotraction, Natchev (1) describes several types of mechanical devices, including the one in Figure 1.1, that have been used over the years for the treatment of back pain. The earliest recorded work-related back injury was 2780 BC (2).

More recently (1858), Virchow and Lushka (3) described the process of intervertebral disc herniation. Interest in the medical world increased dramatically following the famous paper of Mixter and Barr in 1934 (4) describing surgical intervention for the herniated intervertebral disc.

Without question, back pain is one of the most common afflictions that affect modern man. Most authorities familiar with the problem agree that back pain affects nearly 80% of the population in industrialized societies (5). Some studies indicate that one out of every three people has a back problem at any given time (6). In the United States alone it is estimated that back pain affects more than

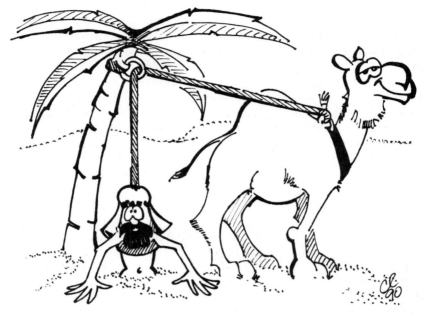

Figure 1.1. Even ancient civilizations developed treatment methods for low back pain. (Adapted from Natchev E. *A manual on autotraction treatment for low back pain.* Sundsvall: Tryckeribolaget, 1984.)

75–80 million individuals (7). Many view the erect bipedal carriage of modern man as the cause of its development or, at the very least, a contributing factor. Others, particularly those involved in industry, view the workplace as the culprit.

Whatever the cause, back pain has become an increasing burden to the health and economy of the industrialized world. Of all the reasons for seeking a doctor's advice, back pain is one of the most common, preceded only by headaches and the common cold. Back pain is a leading cause of work absenteeism. It is the most common cause of disability in persons under the age of 45 and ranks third behind heart disease and arthritis in workers between ages 45 and 64 (8).

While back pain is not usually associated with any life-threatening condition, the costs of the problem are staggering. It has been estimated that the direct costs of back pain in the United States exceed 20 billion dollars per year (9). When indirect costs such as administrating health insurance claims, training new workers to replace a disabled employee, lost productivity, etc. are included, this figure can probably be tripled. Added to these monetary costs are the costs in quality of life for the millions who suffer for long periods of time.

It is stated that low back pain is a "self-limiting condition" that most often goes away in a reasonably short time regardless of the nature of the treatment. Approximately 70% of all back pain will disappear in 3 weeks or less and nearly 90% of back pain patients will feel better within 6–12 weeks. For those suffering from back pain with sciatica the chance of early recovery is not as good but still nearly one out of every two patients will recover within 4 weeks (10). This perception that back pain is "self-limiting" hinders our attempts to control its occurrence.

One of the major premises of this book is that the real problem with back pain is not usually the individual episode. Rather, the problem is: 1) the high rate of recurrence (some estimates place this figure at 95%) (11); 2) the increasing severity of the problem with each recurrence; 3) the small percentage but large numbers of people who suffer for long periods of time; and 4) the relatively young population affected by back pain.

In terms of economic factors, it can be seen that when a patient first suffers an episode of back pain intervention is kept to a minimum. The patient may or may not miss any time at work and usually recovers, as stated earlier, within a few days to a week. With recurrent episodes, however, the patient often seeks help from a physician and may be advised to stay home from work and rest for periods up to 2 weeks. At some point, future episodes may be accompanied by more and more sophisticated evaluation and treatment procedures, including surgery, with more and more time away from work. If, as so often happens, these procedures fail, the patient may eventually end up unable to work and permanently disabled. Obviously the costs for this patient, and for the system that pays the bills, continue to spiral. A second premise of this text is that the system, while established in an attempt to assist the injured worker, in many respects actually adds to the problem.

Although back pain is considered a self-limiting condition for most, approximately 10% of patients with back pain suffer for longer than 3 months. The recovery rate for patients suffering from back pain with sciatica is even lower with approximately 50% suffering more than 1 month (12). Low back pain is seen as the most common cause of disability in workers under age 45. Studies from Great Britain indicate that 1 out of every 25 workers changes jobs because of a back condition (13), and on any given day 0.5% of the work force has been disabled for 6 months or more (14). The individual who is out of work for 6 months has only a 50% chance of returning to work. For those out of work longer than 1 year the likelihood of ever returning to productive employment is only 25%. For greater than 2 years the probability is nil (15).

Several factors combine to make back injuries one of the most costly of all industrial accidents. Back pain affects a largely youthful population with the first episodes most often occurring during the 20s and 30s and a peak in the 40s and 50s (16). Consequently, a worker who is disabled while in his/her 30s or 40s is much more expensive than his/her coworker who is disabled in the late 50s or early 60s as a result of some type of degenerative condition. Each year approximately 500,000 workers have back injuries on the job (17). While most of these recover quickly, the relatively small percentage that does not accounts for the bulk of the costs. Approximately 10–25% of those injured account for 80–90% of the costs (18, 19).

One interesting component of the back pain problem, particularly when considering the injured worker, is that those workers who stand to gain the most from disability or who don't like their work tend to have more severe and more chronic back pain. Beals and Hickman (20) cite several studies to support their contention that therapy that is successful for noncompensated patients is not equally satisfactory for those receiving compensation. Kelsey (21) reported 70.9% of male workers receiving compensation were able to associate a specific task with the onset of low back pain. Only 35.5% of the noncompensated workers made the same association. For female workers the respective percentages were 71.4 and 23.6. As stated earlier, perhaps the very system that is designed to assist the injured worker contributes to the problem.

References

1. Natchev E. *A manual on autotraction treatment for low back pain.* Sundsvall: Tryckeribolaget, 1984.
2. Brandt-Rauf PW, Brandt-Rauf SI. History of occupational medicine: relevance of Imhotep and Edwin Smith papyrus. *Br J Ind Med* 1987;44:68.
3. Virchow R, Luschka HV. *Die Halbgelenke des menschlichen Korpers.* Berlin: Reimer, 1858.
4. Mixter WJ, Barr JS. Rupture of the intervetebral disc with involvement of the spinal canal. *N Engl J Med* 1934;211:210–215.
5. Andersson GBJ, McNeill TW. *Lumbar spine syndromes, evaluation and treatment.* New York: Springer-Verlag, 1989:3.
6. Kirkaldy-Willis WH. *Managing low back pain.* 2nd ed. New York: Churchill-Livingstone, 1988:4.

7. Mandell P, Lipton M, Bernstein J, Kucera G, Kampner J. *Low back pain.* Thorofare, NJ: Slack Inc., 1989:1.
8. Kelsey J, White A, Pastides J, Bisbee G. The impact of musculoskeletal disorders on the population of the United States. *J Bone Joint Surg. Am* 1979;61:959–964.
9. Genant HK. Preface. In: Genant HK, ed. *Spine update 1984: perspectives in radiology, orthopedic surgery, and neurosurgery.* San Francisco: Radiological Research and Education Foundation, 1983.
10. Steinbery GS. *The epidemiology of low back pain.* Stanton-Hicks M, Boas R, eds. New York: Raven Press, 1982:1–12.
11. Steinbery GS. *The epidemiology of low back pain.* Stanton-Hicks M, Boas K, eds. New York: Raven Press, 1982:1–12.
12. Hult L. The Munkfors investigaton. *Acta Orthop Scand* Suppl 1954;16.
13. Pope MH, Frymoyer J, Andersson GBJ. *Occupational low back pain.* New York: Praeger Press, 1984.
14. Wood PHN, Badley EM. Epidemiology of back pain. In: Jayson MI, ed. *The lumbar spine and back pain.* London: Pitman, 1980:13–17.
15. McGill CM. Industrial back problems: a control program. *J Occup Med* 1968;10:174.
16. Biering-Sorensen F. Low back trouble in a general population of 30-, 40-, 50-, and 60-year old men and women. *Dan Med Bull* 1982;29:289–299.
17. National Institute of Occupational Safety and Health. A work practices guide for manual lifting. Technical Report No. 81–122, U. S. Dept. of Health and Human Services (NIOSH), Cincinnati, OH:1981.
18. Spengler DM, Bigos SJ, Martin NA, Zeh J, Fisher L, Nachemson A. Back injuries and industry: a retrospective study. I. Overview and cost analysis. *Spine* 1986;11:241–245.
19. Snook SH. Unpublished data. Hopkinton, MA: Liberty Mutual Insurance, 1987.
20. Beals RK, Hickman NW. Industrial injuries of the back and extremities. *J Bone Joint Surg [Am]* 1972;51A:1593–1611.
21. Kelsey JL. An epidemiological survey of acute herniated lumbar intervertebral discs. *Rheumatol Rehabil* 1975;14:144–159.

2

Classification of Back Pain

In an effort to gain a better understanding of the varied nature of low back pain, a number of classification systems have been developed. While each attempts to address the range of conditions affecting the patient with back pain, it appears that each reflects the individual bias of the author. Some of the more common systems follow.

A. MacNab (1) divided back pain into the following:
1. Viscerogenic
   Kidneys, pelvic viscera, tumors
2. Vascular
   Aneurysms, peripheral vascular disease, intermittent claudication
3. Neurogenic
   CNS tumors, neurofibroma, neurolemmoma, ependymoma
4. Psychogenic
5. Metabolic
6. Spondylogenic
   a. Traumatic lesions
      Infective—pyogenic vertebral osteomyelitis, tuberculosis, miscellaneous infections, intervertebral disc infections, discitis
   b. Neoplastic lesions
      Benign—hemangiomas, medullary islands, osteoid osteoma, osteoblastoma, eosinophilic granuloma, aneurysmal bone cyst, giant cell tumor
   c. Malignant lesions

7

Primary—chordoma, myeloma

Metastatic—most common site

B. McKenzie (2) used the following in his classification of back pain:

1. Postural syndrome—mechanical deformation of postural origin causing pain of a strictly intermittent nature, which appears when the soft tissues surrounding the lumbar segments are placed under prolonged stress

2. Dysfunction syndrome—the condition in which adaptive shortening and resultant loss of mobility causes pain prematurely; this is, before achievement of full normal end range movement

3. Derangement syndrome—internal derangement of the intervertebral disc mechanism

C. Kirkaldy-Willis (3) described the following phases in the degeneration of the lumbar spine:

1. Dysfunction (hypomobility)

Posterior facet syndrome, sacroiliac syndrome, Maigne's syndrome, myofascial syndromes, disc herniation

2. Unstable phase

Facet and disc degeneration, lateral stenosis, central stenosis, disc herniation

3. Stabilization

Lateral stenosis, central stenosis, multilevel stenosis, disc herniation.

In this chapter we will attempt to combine some of the various categories into one single system. We can then look at both the differences and the similarities between each particular category of back pain patient.

Since the focus of this discussion is on the mechanical aspects of back pain it is first helpful to separate into two broad categories: 1) those with some type of nonmechanical disorder (i.e., viscerogenic, vascular, neurogenic, psychogenic, metabolic, infective, and neoplastic); and 2) those resulting from some type of mechanical disorder (spondylogenic). For the purposes of this text we will ignore the various types of back pain with a nonmechanical etiology and cast our attention to those with a mechanical basis. It should be noted, however, that many of the factors that reduce the mechanical type of back pain may also have a positive impact on the nonmechanical patient and good back care should not be ignored in this group.

If we consider those back pain patients with a mechanical spondylogenic disorder we can trace the development and progress of the condition over time. While it is widely accepted that back pain is a self-limiting condition, back problems are not. Rather, in many patients they tend to recur periodically with increasing frequency and severity, often triggered by relatively minor stresses. This increasing problem is frequently seen with a concurrent increase in the degenerative process and an increase in structural findings. By the time these degenerative findings are reflected on the radiographs the patient is often told they have "arthritis" or "disc degeneration" and can expect lifelong problems. Perhaps if early back pain, without obvious structural changes, was seen in a different light preventive steps could be taken to minimize the otherwise inevitable sequelae.

To this end, we will divide those patients with back pain of a mechanical etiology into two subgroups: 1) those with functional pathology and 2) those with structural pathology.

FUNCTIONAL PATHOLOGY

Hans Selye (4) defined disease as "the bodies inability to cope with stress." Health, it seems, is a balance between the inherent coping factors the body possesses and the amount of stress it has to cope with. If we can agree that the human spine is a remarkable engineering accomplishment, we can see that the normal healthy spine can cope with tremendous stresses, provided that it functions properly. Even the healthiest of spines, however, will "break down" if subjected to enough stress for a long enough period of time (see McKenzie's postural syndrome). This prolonged stress may "tip the scale" and result in pain and other symptoms (Fig. 2.1).

If the spine, for whatever reason, fails to function in a smooth, integrated manner then the balance between health and disease may be tipped by lesser amounts of stress. In this instance the problem is not so much the stress but the inadequate ability of the spine to function. This could be seen as the "dysfunction" stage of McKenzie. It is the loss of this smooth, integrated function of each mobile segment, each musculotendinous unit, and each neuromuscular component which may be a primary cause of recurrent problems (back pain). In addition, many consider these functional changes as a primary cause of the degenerative changes that follow.

Unfortunately, the young patient whose symptoms respond readily to treatment is too often considered "well" as soon as such improvement is seen. The underlying functional changes remain and, like a cavity in a tooth, surface when exposed to increasing

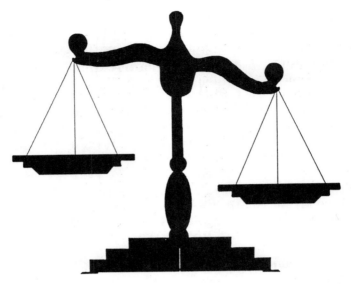

Figure 2.1. Health is a balance between a combination of environmental stressors and the body's ability to cope.

stresses and/or degeneration. Frequently we see the apparently healthy patient told, based on lack of any evident radiographic changes, that there is nothing really wrong. S/he is told to relax and the problem will eventually go away. After all, "back pain is a self-limiting condition."

Chiropractors have long recognized that the status of the vertebral articulations is an important element in spinal health. Early doctors of chiropractic and osteopathy viewed the problem as a "misplaced" vertebra that needed to be restored to its proper position by a manipulation or "adjustment." It is readily apparent, at this point in time, that this lesion involves changes in the mobility and functioning of the vertebral segment. During the early course of the disease such functional changes may not be accompanied by any overt structural changes. Consequently, the physician evaluating the patient is convinced that there is nothing really wrong.

We will divide the "functional" problems into the following categories: (a) articular, (b) myofascial, and (c) neuromuscular. It should be noted that most patients are probably seen with a combination of functional aberrations and that several systems may require evaluation, treatment, and preventive care.

Articular Problems

Mennell (5) was the first to apply the term "dysfunction" to describe the loss of movement commonly known as joint play or accessory movement. Since then other authors have applied the term to articular tissues that are not functioning correctly. McKenzie (6) uses the term to mean "the condition in which adaptive shortening and resultant loss of mobility causes pain prematurely, i.e., before achievement of full normal end range movement." Kirkaldy-Willis (7) has also used the same term to describe the first phase of his "three phases of degeneration" (Phase 1, dysfunction; Phase 2, instability; and Phase 3, stabilization). He states that most patients with low back pain are seen in this phase and that any pathological changes seen are relatively minor and perhaps reversible. He continues that the term "implies that at one anatomical level the three components of the joint are not functioning normally" (7).

The articulations most directly associated with the onset of back pain are the posterior lumbosacral facets, the sacroiliac joints, and the posterior facets of the upper lumbar and thoraco-lumbar spine. In addition, since the spine functions as a closed kinematic chain, improper functioning of other spinal levels, such as the upper cervical segments, should be included. Also, attention must be directed at the functioning of the hip joints and the other joints of the lower kinetic chain.

Posterior Facet Syndrome

During the early phase of this syndrome the patient may present with a localized unilateral back pain that may or may not be accompanied by leg pain. The clinical appearance may be remarkably similar to the patient with intervertebral disc (IVD) disease and an accurate delineation between the two may not be possible. It would appear that the nature of the factors that aggravate or relieve the symptoms might be most helpful in determining the precise location of the lesion. (Note: while each of these syndromes are described and discussed separately it is my opinion that they rarely exist alone. In most patients the objective observer will find an assortment of functional disturbances that individually or collectively produce symptoms.)

It is suggested that a patient with an early posterior facet syndrome would likely be more comfortable in a slightly forward, bent posture while standing or sitting. (The increase in intra-discal pressure seen in the seated position seems often to aggravate many disc lesions.) Backward bending, on the other hand, brings the facet articulations into a close-packed position, a position of maximal neuronal activity. It could be safely assumed that this would aggravate an inflamed facet and increase symptoms.

As already discussed, in the early stages of a posterior facet syndrome there may be a marked functional alteration and yet no identifiable structural changes. Consequently, the patient with an early posterior facet syndrome may appear completely normal on x-ray, magnetic resonance, or computerized tomography. The most reliable means of localizing the lesion may be the subjective changes associated with palpation of movement and local tissue texture changes. It would appear that, even after the pain and symptoms have resolved, these functional changes should still be identifiable and will likely continue to trigger future attacks of back pain when sufficiently provoked.

Sacroiliac Syndrome

Perhaps one of the most misunderstood articulations in the human body is the sacroiliac joint. Even less understood is the role of the sacroiliac (SI) joint in the developement of back pain. The joint serves to transfer the weight of the head, arms, and trunk to the lower limbs. It possesses a small amount of movement, perhaps 3–5 degrees in the child, but appears to gradually stiffen during the first 4–5 decades, which is associated with a gradual fibrosis of the joint.

The sacroiliac joint is an extremely stable articulation, perhaps the strongest in the spine. It is secured by strong, well-developed ligaments and, at best, is only slightly mobile. It would appear that instability or even hypermobility would be most unlikely in this joint. It would also appear that any reduction of its relatively small amount of movement would not have a dramatic impact on other functions of the spine. And yet, doctors of chiropractic and osteopathy, physical therapists, and others familiar with manual manipulative procedures have long recognized the often dramatic symptomatic and functional changes seen with SI joint manipulation. It is not clear how dysfunction of this joint causes pain. Perhaps pain may be associated with muscle spasm and/or reflex muscular changes. It seems unlikely that pain is primarily due to the joint itself. Likewise, the exact mechanism to explain the clinical changes seen has not yet been adequately described.

The patient with a sacroiliac syndrome will often present with a localized pain over the SI joint, often unilateral. This may or may not be associated with leg pain. Pain is felt directly over the joint and may be present while standing and walking and relieved by sitting. Patients often complain of difficulty rising from a chair only to find relief after taking a few steps. Many also experience an increase in local pain while climbing stairs.

Many of the exercises found in back exercise programs affect the flexibility of the sacroiliac joint (knees to chest, leg raises, toe-touches, flexion-extension on all fours, etc.), which may help to explain the benefits of such exercises.

Posterior Facet Syndrome of Upper Lumbar and Thoraco-lumbar Spine (Maigne's Syndrome)

Since the spine functions as a closed kinematic chain, if any portion of the chain fails to function normally the entire unit is affected. A chain typically breaks at its "weakest link" and it has been recognized by chiropractors for many years that, while the low back may be the area of pain, other areas of the spine can contribute to the problem and may actually cause the condition. Such an example would be Maigne's syndrome. This condition is associated with pain supplying the skin at the level of the iliac crest and may or may not be accompanied by pain localized to the lower back and buttocks. Manipulation of the thoraco-lumbar junction has been seen, by this author, to remedy the painful situation, often with dramatic and immediate results.

While it is not too difficult for the individual unfamiliar with manipulative procedures to envision a relationship between a dysfunction in the thoraco-lumbar spine and lower back pain, perhaps one of the most confusing and controversial aspects of manual medicine is the relationship between more cephalad segments of the spine and lower back pain. If we can rely on clinical evidence it would seem that some patients presenting with pain localized in the lower back respond most effectively to manipulation of the cervical spine, especially the upper cervical segments. Lewit (8) describes a group of school-age children with pelvic dysfunction and a high incidence of accompanying suboccipital lesions. With manipulation of the suboccipital spine the pelvic distortion was said to disappear.

Once again, the exact mechanisms for this response is not clear. Perhaps the change is strictly mechanical and can be explained using the principles of dysfunction in the kinematic chain. Or perhaps the change is more a neuromuscular phenomenon and relates to a reflex change either in muscular tension and/or neuromuscular control of the kinematic chain. Regardless of the explanation, it should be borne in mind that the patient with low back pain is not "just another low back" but a complex individual who must be viewed in his/her entirety (Fig. 2.2).

Hip-Spine Syndrome

Concurrent disease at both the hip and the spine is not infrequent, particularly in the elderly population, and is referred to as hip-spine syndrome. Offierski and MacNab (9) describe a simple hip-spine syndrome in which there is only one source of disability, either the hip or the spine, and a complex hip-spine syndrome in which symptomatic changes may be derived from both hip and spine.

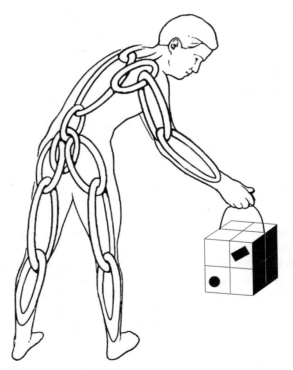

Figure 2.2. The musculoskeletal system is a series of "kinematic chains." (Adapted from Mayer TG, Gatchel RJ. *Functional restoration for spinal disorders: the sports medicine approach*. Philadelphia: Lea & Febiger, 1984.)

The participation of the hip joint in the function of the lower back was clearly described by Cailliett (10) in his description of the lumbar-pelvic rhythm. This is defined as the ratio between two movements occurring simultaneously in one plane (lumbar spine movement and pelvic rotation). The act of bending forward to touch the floor or pick up a pencil would not be possible without the contribution of the hip joints. It must be assumed that any change in the smooth functioning of the hip joint or any disruption in this lumbar-pelvic rhythm must be adapted for. It is reasonable to see that a partial loss of hip movement will increase the stress and loads on the lumbosacral portion of the rhythm and may easily trigger the progression of changes leading to low back pain.

The patient with an acetabular syndrome may present with a primary complaint of pain in the lower back and buttocks. The appearance may be remarkably similar to the patient with a disc syndrome. One patient seen by this author had an apparent "textbook case" of sciatic radiculitis with radiation of pain and symptoms consistent with such a condition. She had been seen by six different physicians of varying specialties. Each had diagnosed an intervertebral disc syndrome accompanied by sciatica and had treated the lumbosacral spine accordingly. To the patient's frustration, however, the problem had persisted for nearly 6 years with little relief. Upon examination, marked reduction in acetabular mobility was seen and a course of mobilization, manipulation, and exercise for the hip joint was instituted. Within 5 weeks the patient was free of pain and able to resume a normal productive life.

While the patient with an acetabular syndrome may appear similar to the other low back patients two points will be evident: 1) pain and tenderness over the greater trochanter, and 2) limitation of acetabular movement. This movement limitation may be identified with Patrick-Fabers test, heel-to-buttocks test, and in lack of pelvic rotation with forward bending of the trunk. It can be assumed that, in addition to altering the lumbosacral movement patterns, acetabular dysfunction may also trigger sacroiliac changes that may be inaccurately diagnosed as SI syndrome. As with the sacroiliac joint, many of the exercises traditionally performed for back pain are seen to increase the mobility of the hip.

Dysfunction in the Lower Chain

One of the functions of the lumbar spine, particularly the intervertebral disc, is to serve as a shock absorber for the remainder of the spine. This shock-absorbing function is also served by the joints of the lower limbs such as the knee, ankle, and foot. A change in the ability of these joints to adequately perform this function may overload the lumbar spine and contribute to the development of lower back pain. When the chiropractic physician is confronted with the low back pain patient who is unresponsive, evaluation of these shock-absorbing mechanisms may be appropriate. Treatment may include manipulation, exercises, foot orthotics, or podiatric referral.

In addition to aiding the shock-absorbing mechanisms of the spine the lower limb also functions, in conjunction with the hip joint, in another closed kinematic chain. If we conclude that dysfunction in one part of a closed chain may trigger malfunction in other parts of the same chain we must also recognize that dysfunction in one chain may exert increasing demands on other adjacent chains. The hip-knee-ankle represents a closed kinematic chain. Perhaps dysfunction of the ankle might so distort this lower chain that the function of the hip is affected. This, in turn, might affect the lumbar-pelvic rhythm and manifest as lower back pain.

The possibilities are seemingly endless and we could continue with this discussion indefinitely. Suffice it to say that the patient with lower back pain may have many contributing factors that individually or collectively create a state of unrest in the lumbar spine. Not all patients with low back pain require treatment or rehabilitation directed at the painful area. The chiropractor must be constantly alert to the subtleties of the individual and remain "open" to the possibilities.

Myofascial Problems

According to Kirkaldy-Willis (11) six different myofascial syndromes are associated with low back pain. In actual fact, there are probably many more. He describes a cycle of events that include emotional factors, changes in muscles, and changes in the components of the three joint complex. It is often seen that the onset of back pain is preceded by a period of increased stress and tension (both physical and emotional) (Fig. 2.3).

It is most likely that changes in the muscle do not occur in isolation to changes in the joint and vice versa. Rather, the myofascial cycle may be used to understand the interaction between the various tissues. With normal use muscle tissue is continually contracting and relaxing and adapting to varying demands. During certain situations, however, such as prolonged postural stress, the

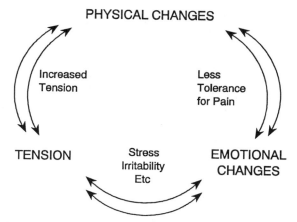

Figure 2.3. Back pain is often preceded by increased stress and tension. (Adapted from Mayer TG, Gatchel RJ. *Functional restoration for spinal disorders: the sports medicine approach.* Philadelphia: Lea & Febiger, 1984.)

muscle tissue may contract for long periods of time without adequate periods of rest. The result of this prolonged contraction is tightening of the muscle and a build-up of toxins and waste products in the muscle and surrounding tissues. With this comes a constriction of blood vessels necessary to supply nutrients to the muscle and carry waste products away. Added to this may be an assortment of emotional stresses that exacerbate the problem (Fig. 2.4).

With a continuing load, such as might be found on the work-site where an employee is forced to stand in an awkward position for extended periods at a time, day after day, these changes in the muscle may become more and more fixed. This increase in muscle tension may be recognized in changes in joint function or hypomobility of associated joints.

Rather than being primary, the changes occurring in the muscle may be secondary to the joint changes. If a joint is immobilized for a period of time, the muscles associated with the joint will atrophy. This is seen in muscle wasting during orthopedic casting procedures. It would appear that partial changes in mobility might also lead to changes in muscle function and tone, but to a lesser degree. Regardless of the etiology of the muscular changes, the net result is often an increase in muscle tone, or hypertonus. This may be viewed as a dysfunction of the muscle, akin to the joint dysfunction discussed earlier.

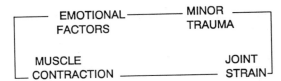

Figure 2.4. The relationship between emotions and trauma to low back pain. (Adapted from Kirkaldy-Willis WH. *Managing low back pain,* 2nd ed. New York: Churchill-Livingstone, 1988.)

Janda (12) describes five different types of muscular changes each with its own characteristics and appearance:

1. Those attributable to increased activity of the limbic system, i.e., stress. These are seen as a generalized increase in muscle tension that affects an entire region of the body such as the lower back, or neck and shoulder region.
2. Those attributable to segmental joint restriction and the accompanying neurological irritation, i.e., the chiropractic subluxation complex, or Korr's facilitated segment. These are often seen to be unilateral and may follow the course of a peripheral nerve supply.
3. Those associated with viscero-somatic reflexes. An example is the lower back pain and muscle spasms associated with urinary tract infections. These are often regional and bilateral and accompanied by an elevation of temperature and other systemic findings.
4. Those associated with the development of myofascial trigger points. These are typically localized to a single muscle and predictable in location.
5. Those associated simply with disuse and shortening such as the shortened hamstrings in a sedentary person. These changes often fit into relatively common muscular patterns, the upper and lower crossed syndromes described in Chapter 3.

A familiarization with the myofascial syndromes presented in *Myofascial Pain and Dysfunction* by Travell and Simons would be most helpful at this point. Kirkaldy-Willis (13) describes syndromes associated with the gluteus medius and maximus, the piriformis, the quadratus lumborum, the tensor fasciae latae, and the hamstrings. In reality, many more myofascial syndromes present with low back pain. The treatment often involves methods directed at the myofascial tissues, and prevention involves both stretching exercises and elimination or reduction or postural stresses, particularly those on the job.

Neuromuscular Problems

Included under this heading are problems of balance and coordination as well as altered patterns of movement and problems with proprioception. It is not common practice to include such problems in a textbook about back pain, but recent developments in the treatment of many different musculoskeletal problems, including back pain, have seen an increasing interest in the evaluation and rehabilitation of these aspects. The use of the BAPS board, the wobble board, and other similar apparatus are examples of attempts to improve proprioception, balance, and coordination.

Serious athletes have known for years that proper balance and coordination are vital to the proper performance of specific activities. One only has to consider the downhill skier or the Olympic gymnast to realize the importance. The injured worker that Gilliam (14) refers to as "the industrial athlete" is equally dependent upon proper balance and coordination in order to perform his/her daily activities.

It is accepted that an injury such as a sprained ankle will often result in a loss of strength and range of motion of the affected appendage. This may last long after the pain and swelling have disappeared and may contribute to the incidence of future injuries. The athlete often complains of the ankle "giving out" at the least provocation. Less well appreciated is the loss or change in proprioception, balance, and coordination. To demonstrate this change one only has to ask the individual with chronic ankle or knee problems to balance on one leg with eyes closed. Deprived of any visual assistance, this is accomplished easily only when the body is supplied with adequate proprioceptive input from the joints and muscles. Any distortion of the input from the joint and muscle proprioceptors can be seen by a noticeable loss of balance. This is often dramatic from one limb to the other and serves to reinforce the need for rehabilitation in this area.

It can be assumed that alterations in spinal joint and muscle function may also be associated with changes in proprioceptive input. Since the body is continually attempting to adapt to variations in signal input, the more accurate the incoming information, the more likely the adaptive response is appropriate.

Specific exercises aimed at improving muscle coordination and balance will be described in Chapter 6.

STRUCTURAL PATHOLOGY

One of the principal tenets of the chiropractic profession is the direct relationship between structure and function. Those conditions, originally presenting as primarily functional in nature, in time will develop structural changes. Kirkaldy-Willis (3) discusses the degenerative process in the three phases of degeneration. It has become increasingly more accepted that the degenerative process may indeed be triggered by functional changes and that early identification and correction of these functional changes may delay or even prevent its otherwise inevitable progression (16).

With continued functional pathology whether it be articular, myofascial, neuromuscular, or a combination, it can be shown that structural changes will ensue. Many authors have considered the normal functioning of the musculoskeletal structures to be a key element in the very longevity of the tissues (16). Kessler and Hertling (15) state that "although it is recognized that mechanical changes also occur, these are usually not dealt with until advanced structural changes have resulted. The earlier, conservative treatment in joint disease typically involves measures to counter the physiological changes taking place. . . . It is well accepted that joint disease may result from some mechanical disturbance . . . although it has been postulated by some that primary osteoarthrosis has a physiologic or metabolic etiology, it appears that in many cases it is due to mechanical changes."

Kirkaldy-Willis (3) describes the progression from dysfunction or hypomobility to degeneration of the facet articulations and the intervertebral disc. With further insult, further degeneration occurs, sometimes resulting in disruption and instability.

Articular Problems

Posterior Facet Syndrome

The changes seen in the articulations of the spine in this phase are best described by Kirkaldy-Willis and include narrowing of the joint space, thinning of the articular cartilage, and osteophyte formation (3). These changes may be dramatic and show clearly on plain film radiography as well as magnetic resonance and computerized tomography scan. There is little doubt that these changes affect the low back patient. The puzzling part is the individual with marked degenerative changes who has no back pain. In addition, the patient who presents with marked degenerative changes associated with back pain whose symptoms disappear only to be left with the same marked degenerative changes. Consequently, the correlation between osteoarthrosis and back pain is not clear.

Treatment should be directed at the functional changes associated with the condition. Hypomobility may be improved by mobilizing procedures and manipulation in addition to stretching exercises. Instability may be reduced by improving the function of other parts of the kinematic chain and by strengthening exercises.

Sacroiliac Syndrome

As mentioned earlier, the sacroiliac joint appears to lose much of its mobility with advancing age. This is usually accompanied by a gradual fibrosis and sometimes by calcification of the joint. Whether this is a natural aging process or simply the result of a decreasing demand on the joint common with decreasing activity is unclear. Marked degenerative changes in this joint are seldom seen in the absence of systemic disease such as ankylosing spondylitis.

Posterior Facet Syndrome of Upper Lumbar and Thoraco-lumbar Spine

Degenerative changes similar to those described with the lower lumbar facets may also occur at other levels of the spine. These may often go unrecognized and certainly may not be associated with the patient's painful lower back. It is suggested that advancing degenerative changes at these levels may be associated with an increasing demand on lumbosacral tissues and may contribute to the development of instability at these levels. Improvement of function at these upper lumbar spinal segments will often lessen the demand on the lumbosacral tissues and can be seen to improve the symptom picture.

Hip-Spine Syndrome

Marked degenerative changes in the hip joint often need to occur in order to gain the attention of the physician. The patient is often told that s/he has arthritis or bursitis of the hip and is given medication to relieve the discomfort. It appears that only when the degeneration is complete is an attempt made to remedy the situation and an implant is performed. Several studies linking the incidence of back pain and degeneration of the hip joint appear in the literature. Friberg (16) claims that, while the condition is typically associated with aging, it is actually seen early in life, long before radiologic signs of degenerative diseases appear. I have long suspected a relationship. As with the facet articulations, the degenerative process follows that of any other synovial joint and includes reduction in joint space, thinning of articular cartilage, and reactive bone formation and spurring.

Dysfunction in the Lower Chain

We may associate the advancing degenerative changes described here with any synovial joint in the body, including those in the lower limb. The difficulty remains in linking these changes to continuing degeneration in the spine. While ample evidence exists to develop reasonable hypotheses, the connection remains speculative.

Spinal Stenosis

The reactive degenerative changes may reach dramatic proportions in the development of spinal stenosis, both lateral and central. Perhaps no one single degenerative condition has the potential for more symptom changes than this. The progression of changes involves degeneration of both facets and intervertebral disc (IVD), loss of disc height, subluxation of facets with encroachment of the inferior facet on the pedicle above, narrowing of the intervertebral foramen (IVF), and eventual entrapment of the spinal nerve (17). The patient may or may not complain of back pain. Pain is frequently seen in the buttocks, the hip, or the sciatic distribution. Pain may extend into the calf to the foot. The patient may complain of symptoms of nerve compression such as paraesthesia or sensory loss. Since forward bending of the spine opens the IVF, flexion often provides some relief. Symptoms may be aggravated by activity and patients may be unable to find a comfortable position.

Central stenosis may have a similar appearance with one or both limbs affected and motor weakness the predominant symptom (23). The symptom picture may be confusing with multiple levels affected. Walking may be very difficult (neurogenic claudication). Bicycle riding, on the other hand, with the lumbar spine in flexion, is not painful.

Radiographs demonstrate marked changes, including enlarged posterior facets, decreased interlaminar distance, decreased distance between the articular processes, diminished disc height, vertebral body osteophytes, and reduction in size of the IVF.

Intervertebral Disc Syndrome

No single structure in the low back has received more attention than the intervertebral disc. While there is some disagreement regarding the exact percentages, most agree that many low back patients do indeed suffer some type of IVD syndrome. Cyriax (24) attributed most lumbar spine pain to internal derangement of the IVD mechanism. McKenzie (25) claimed that as many as 95% of his patients have IVD problems. Williams (26) stated emphatically "The bottom disc has ruptured in the majority of all persons by the age of 20 years . . ." Andersson (27) states that the claims of a high frequency of discogenic back pain are supported by "circumstantial evidence, pathological studies, biomechanical studies, experimental studies, etc."

Regardless of the precise numbers or mechanisms, the role of the intervertebral disc in the production of low back pain, with or without leg pain, is indisputed. Since Mixter and Barr (28) described the IVD as a source of pain in 1934, a number of different, and sometimes conflicting, methods of evaluation and treatment have developed based on the particular observations of the individual author. If we look at the role of the IVD, the aging process, and the types of mechanical insult to which the disc is subjected, we can begin to decipher this confusing structure.

The IVD is a unique structure in the human body. Classified as a ligament it serves, in part, to hold the spinal column together. Structured unlike any other ligament it also, simultaneously, serves to hold the vertebral bodies apart. Its principal tasks, however, are to serve as a shock-absorbing mechanism for the spine and to facilitate movement between the vertebrae.

In the young healthy spine the IVD, being largely water, serves its combined functions well. As we age, however, the very structure of the disc changes and its ability to function changes with it. As part of the three-joint complex, any change in IVD function is seen to directly affect the functioning of the posterior facets and vice versa.

The disc begins life with a large centrally placed acellular nucleus pulposus that is approximately 90% fluid. The surrounding annulus fibrosus is only 80% fluid and there seems to be a clear delineation between nucleus and annulus. Very early in life the disc loses its sparse blood supply and by the second decade is said to be largely avascular. In fact, the IVD is often described as the largest avascular structure in the body. The significance of this early loss of blood supply lies in the reduced ability of the disc to repair itself when injured. In addition, since the disc is basically a hydraulic mechanism, its ability to adapt to changing internal pressures may be diminished. Any nutrients brought to the disc and any waste products removed occurs via a fluid exchange that takes place across the cartilage end plates of the vertebral body.

As pressure increases, fluid must pass through the end plates into the vertebral body and as pressure decreases the reverse occurs. This exchange acts as a safety valve to reduce the likelihood of dangerous increases in internal pressure.

In addition to a decrease in the vascular supply, several other important changes occur in the disc with aging that must be considered. There is a gradual desiccation, drying, or loss of fluid that is seen. By the third decade the nucleus is said to be approximately 80% fluid and the annulus roughly 75%. With advancing years the fluid content of the nucleus is decreased to slightly more than 70% with the annulus slightly less. In other words, the delineation between nucleus pulposus and annulus fibrosus gradually is lost to the point where it may become difficult to tell one from the other. Saunders (29) describes this as a transition from chewing gum to crabmeat.

Obviously the mechanical properties of the aged disc are markedly different from that of the teenager. It is no surprise that discogenic back pain seems to peak at a relatively young age (45–60) only to be replaced by back pain more consistent with degenerative changes in the three-joint complex, i.e., stenosis.

The IVD is a viscoelastic structure and, as such, is subject to creep deformation and hysteresis. Creep deformation is defined as a deformation that occurs over time. Both Williams and McKenzie alluded to this creep deformation that occurs with prolonged postural stresses, although each saw it through slightly different lenses. Williams (30) claimed that lumbar extension was a counterproductive posture due to its effect on the IVD and issued his "First Commandment for low back and leg pain sufferers: always sit, stand, walk, and lie in a way that reduces the hollow of the low back to a minimum." McKenzie (31), on the other hand, holds that a continued decrease in lumbar extension so loads the posterior aspect of the IVD that disc degeneration is almost inevitable. Perhaps either posture sustained over a prolonged time allows the disc to gradually deform and contributes to its demise.

Hysteresis is defined as a gradual loss of energy with repetitive load and unload cycles. The disc, subjected to sustained repetitive impact, such as that which occurs with an over-the-road truck driver or a farmer driving a tractor, gradually fatigues. It is no coincidence that such occupations have a high incidence of disco-genic back pain.

The aging process in the IVD involves a gradual loss of fluid and shock-absorbing capacity. In addition, with trauma, the annulus begins to split and crack. This is first seen in the development of concentric tears that we may speculate are consistent with MacNab's "protrusion" (32) and may occur along with early, self-healing episodes of back pain. These cracks allow swelling in the discal tissues with, perhaps, temporary pain. With increasing trauma comes a coalescence of the tears and the development of radial tears. It would appear that this could be correlated with an increasing frequency and intensity of pain that is consistent with the history of the "typical back patient." With this internal disruption comes a loss of disc height, increasing stresses on the posterior facets and the concomitant degenerative joint disease.

Too often, disc problems are viewed as having an immediate onset. The worker bends over to lift a box, hears a "pop" in his/her back, and complains of pain. Lifting the box is probably only the last step in a series of degenerative steps, much like the cavity in the tooth that is noticed upon biting into an apple.

Mennell (33) lists a series of criteria that he felt were necessary for the diagnosis of IVD disease:

1. A history of trauma severe enough to injure an intact disc;
2. A history of low back pain;
3. A history of secondary trauma, insufficient to injure an intact disc but adequate to disrupt an already weakened disc.

If we evaluate these criteria in light of the changes taking place in the disc and the typical back pain patient, things begin to add up.

THE "TYPICAL PATIENT"

My interest in low back pain stems, in part, from my own personal experience as a back pain patient. My first recollection of back pain was at the age of 18. I was employed as a sacker in a grocery store and hurt my low back while pushing a customer's car out of a snow-covered parking lot. A few days later I visited our family doctor only to be told that if the pain did not go away in 1 week we'd look into it. As luck would have it, I awoke several days later completely free of pain. No attempt was made to determine the cause or nature of my pain and both the doctor and myself assumed that I was "well." (After all, back pain is a self-limiting condition.) Over the years I have had several acute episodes of back pain, the worst occurring after helping a friend carry a heavy table down a flight of stairs. Each time the onset appeared to involve flexion of my lumbar spine. I learned that back bending was a most helpful procedure for my back and consequently incorporated McKenzie's protocols in the treatment of many of my patients. While the incident in the parking lot was the first time that I knew my back was injured, in retrospect I recalled having a rather serious accident on a toboggan some 10 years earlier. I have often wondered if there was a correlation between the two injuries; perhaps this fit Mennell's criteria. My frustration with my back pain increased with each new episode and I decided to learn how to avoid new injuries.

DISC HERNIATIONS

MacNab (34) classifies the various categories of intervertebral disc herniations as follows:

A. Disc protrusion—a localized bulge of the annulus with no disruption of fibers; probably short-lived symptoms.
B. Disc herniations—involves some type of disruption of annular fibers. The following type of herniations are seen:
   1. Vertical herniation—nuclear material bursts through the vertebral body endplates. This probably occurs at a young age when the disc is highly fluid-filled and the vertebral endplates are soft. The injury is thought to be due to a compressive force such as a "pratfall" and may result in the development of Schmorl's nodes.
   2. Horizontal herniation—the most common variety seen in the adult may be central, medial, or lateral.
      a. Prolapse—disruption of internal annular fibers with the outer fibers remaining intact. This may be seen to be consistent with the development of the tears seen in many aging discs.
      b. Extrusion—involves disruption of both internal and external annular fibers. The displaced nuclear fluid is held in its position by the outer ligaments of the spine.
      c. Sequestration—nuclear material bursts through the annular fibers and the outer spinal ligaments and lies within the spinal canal. Mennell (35) refers to this type of herniation as an "epidural tumor."

It is clear that problems in the IVD do, under certain circumstances, cause pain. It is not clear, however, exactly how the disc produces such pain. The IVD must be considered as a contributor to the development of back pain and not as the "cause of the problem." Care must be taken to avoid viewing the disc as the culprit.

SUMMARY

The differential diagnosis of low back pain remains, to this day, a controversial topic. Specialists do not always agree on the precise nature of the lesion or on the necessary treatment. Whether a particular patient suffers from discogenic back pain or from some type of malady of the posterior facets may be debated, ad nauseam. In the long run, however, it may not be all that important. I am of the opinion that patients do not present with an intervertebral disc syndrome that has developed in isolation from the remainder of the body, nor do they present with a posterior facet that is the only structure impacted. They present with complex problems that collectively, not individually, affect this important structure.

Even when agreement is reached regarding the nature of the condition, the treatment varies considerably from doctor to doctor even within the same specialty. Saunders (36) states that doctors tend to treat based on their training and philosophy rather than on the nature of the condition. The general practitioner tends to treat with pain relievers, muscle relaxants, and bed rest. The chiropractor manipulates. The physical therapist is directed to apply heat, ultrasound, and traction, and the surgeon looks for something to remove or repair.

Seldom is the patient evaluated in his/her entirety. It is imperative that each doctor who chooses to accept the responsibility of caring for a patient with a low back problem view the patient in the context presented in this text. That is, full attention should be paid to each patient's lifestyle, environment at home as well as on the job, general physical and mental health, social environment, etc. In addition, each patient must learn to accept the simple fact that any long term change in the condition of their back is largely up to them. To do any less is unacceptable.

References

1. MacNab I. *Backache.* Baltimore: Williams & Wilkins, 1977:17–18.
2. McKenzie R. *The lumbar spine: mechanical diagnosis and therapy.* Wellington, New Zealand: Spinal Publications, 1985.
3. Kirkaldy-Willis WH, ed. *Managing low back pain,* 2nd ed. New York: Churchill-Livingstone, 1988:117–131.

4. Selye H, *Stress without distress*. Philadelphia: J.B. Lippincott, 1974.
5. Mennell JM, *Joint pain*. Boston: Little, Brown, 1964.
6. McKenzie R. *The lumbar spine: mechanical diagnosis and therapy*. Wellington, New Zealand: Spinal Publications, 1985:95.
7. Kirkaldy-Willis WH, ed. *Managing low back pain*, 2nd ed. New York: Churchill-Livingstone, 1988:117.
8. Lewit K. *Manipulative therapy in rehabilitation of the locomotor system*. London: Butterworth, 1988:26–27.
9. Offierski CM, MacNab I. Hip-spine syndrome. *Spine* 1983;8(3):316–321.
10. Cailliett R. *Low back pain syndromes*, 2nd ed. Philadelphia: F.A. Davis, 1968:23–26.
11. Kirkaldy-Willis WH, ed. *Managing low back pain*, 2nd ed. New York: Churchill-Livingstone, 1988:138–141.
12. Janda MIV. Lecture Series, Los Angeles College of Chiropractic, 1989.
13. Kirkaldy-Willis WH, ed. *Managing low back pain*, 2nd ed. New York: Churchill-Livingstone, 1988:138–141.
14. Gilliam T. Lecture, Cybex Seminar, San Diego, 1989.
15. Kessler RM, Hertling D. *Management of common musculoskeletal disorders*. Philadelphia: Harper and Row, 1983:11–49.
16. Salter R. *Textbook of disorders and injuries of the musculoskeletal system*, 2nd ed. Baltimore: Williams & Wilkins, 1983:30–37.
21. Friberg O. Hip-spine syndrome; Clinical biomechanics, diagnosis, and conservative treatment. *Manual Med.* 1988;3:144–147.
22. Kirkaldy-Willis WH, ed. *Managing low back pain*, 2nd ed. New York: Churchill-Livingstone, 1988:144.
23. Kirkaldy-Willis WH, ed. *Managing low back pain*, 2nd ed. New York: Churchill-Livingstone, 1988:148.
24. Cyriax J. *Textbook of Orthopaedic Medicine*. Vol. 1; Diagnosis of soft tissue lesions. London: Bailliere Tendall, 1982.
25. McKenzie R. *The lumbar spine: mechanical diagnosis and therapy*. Wellington, New Zealand: Spinal Publications, 1985:109.
26. Williams PC. *Low back and neck pain: causes and conservative treatment*. Springfield: Charles C. Thomas, 1974.
27. Andersson GBJ, McNeill TW, *Lumbar spine syndromes, evaluation and treatment*. New York: Springer-Verlag, 1989:23.
28. Mixter WJ, Barr JS. Rupture of the intervertebral disc with involvement of the spinal canal. *N Engl J Med*. 1934;211:210–215.
29. Saunders HD. *Evaluation, treatment and prevention of musculoskeletal disorders*. Minneapolis: Viking Press, 1985:305.
30. Williams PC. *Low back and neck pain, causes and conservative treatment*. Springfield: Charles C. Thomas, 1974:20.
31. McKenzie R. *The lumbar spine: mechanical diagnosis and therapy*. Wellington, New Zealand: Spinal Publications, 1985:81.
32. MacNab I. *Backache*. Baltimore: Williams and Wilkins, 1977:92.
33. Mennell JM, *Back Pain*. Boston: Little, Brown, 1960:64.
34. MacNab I. *Backache*. Baltimore: Williams and Wilkins, 1977:91–93.
35. Mennell JM, *Back Pain*. Boston: Little, Brown, 1960:64.
36. Saunders HD, *Evaluation, treatment and prevention of musculoskeletal disorders*. Minneapolis: Viking Press, 1985:305.

3

Causes of Low Back Pain

While the problem of lower back pain is almost universal in dimension, the underlying mechanisms that lead to such pain are not agreed upon. Whether the intervertebral disc, the facet articulations, the ligaments, the myofascial structures, or other tissues are primarily at fault is rarely clear and often subject to the individual interpretation and bias of the examiner. Regardless of the differential diagnosis, we can separate low back pain into that which is mechanical or nonpathological in nature and that which is related to some type of pathological process as was described in the previous chapter. For the purposes of this discussion we will consider only the mechanical type of back pain.

It has been recognized for some time that factors present in our environment influence the prevalence of back pain. Fahrni (1) saw a reduced frequency in ground-dwelling populations. He noted that such population groups maintained a flexed posture throughout the day and concluded that the maintenance of such a flexed posture would reduce the incidence of low back pain and intervertebral disc degeneration. Williams (2) made similar observations and used this to develop his flexion exercise program. These exercises are used to reduce the lumbar lordosis and flatten the lumbar spine. This exercise protocol has been used for many years as a standard exercise regimen for back pain patients. (The Williams flexion exercises will be described later in Chapter 6.)

McKenzie (3), on the other hand, felt that widespread low back pain is due to "an almost universal loss of extension." He developed a treatment regimen and exercise protocol with the express intent of recreating the lumbar lordosis. (McKenzie's exercise protocol will be described in Chapter 6.) As with the Williams flexion exercises,

McKenzie's extension protocol has become widely accepted and is practiced throughout the world.

With such contradictory information it seems difficult indeed to reach any firm conclusions regarding the etiology of low back pain. Even though Williams and McKenzie saw the development of back pain through very different lenses, they both felt that factors in the individual's environment could positively or negatively influence the problem. We will attempt, in this chapter, to look at the similarities in patients with back problems.

Rather than search for a single, isolated factor that is *the* cause of back pain it is perhaps more useful to view back pain in the same manner that we view other degenerative conditions such as heart disease, i.e., the end-product of years of improper habits and abuse. Consider the 45-year-old office worker who suffers a heart attack while mowing the lawn. After initial intervention aimed at saving his life his condition is explained to him by the cardiologist. He is told that mowing the lawn did not "cause" his heart condition. Rather, it merely triggered the attack. His heart problem is the result of years of abuse including stress, a terrible diet, high blood pressure, weight problems, and a lack of regular exercise. He is told, in no uncertain terms, that his health is in his hands and that such continued abuse and disregard for his body will have a predictable outcome. Whether or not the patient elects to change his lifestyle and take charge of his health, he at least understands that he, and only he, can solve the problem.

Next, consider a similar 45-year-old office worker who hurts his back while pulling the chain to start his lawnmower. Rather than view his condition as the result of years of abuse and neglect, he prefers to blame the lawnmower. When he seeks care for his condition he assumes that the doctor will solve his problems for him with a "magic potion, pill, or crack of the back." How often have we heard the patient describe several similar episodes in the past. He may even state that he has sought assistance before, perhaps from another chiropractor. Too often he assumes that, since he only recently developed pain, his back problem must be a recent development also. Once the pain is gone, so the back problem must be gone. This belief is too often reinforced by the physician.

Regardless of the specific type of mechanical back pain and the particular environmental factors that contribute to its continuation we can reasonably assume that the following factors are individually or collectively associated with its development (4):

1. Posture
2. Improper daily habits
3. Poor body mechanics
4. Loss of flexibility
5. Reduced levels of fitness
6. Stress

Recognizing that there is *no single* cause of back pain is a major step in reducing its prevalence and is one of the most important concepts that needs to be relayed in any patient education program (Fig. 3.1).

1. POSTURE

One of the common factors in the daily activities of industrialized societies is the maintenance of a flexed, forward-bent posture. Picture, if you will, the typical day of an office worker. S/he arises

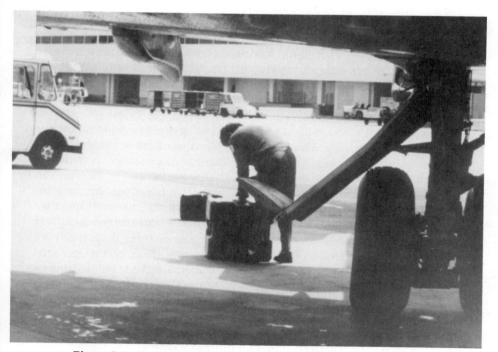

Figure 3.1. Back pain is the result of an accumulation of stresses.

early in the morning and sits at the breakfast table bent over the morning paper. Following breakfast s/he gets in the family car and drives 30 minutes to work, again in a flexed, forward-bent position. Once at work, s/he sits at a desk for the next 8 hours. The afternoon commute home sees our office worker in the same flexed position. After eating the evening meal s/he sits in a relaxed position to watch a couple of hours of television. In a typical day it is rare that s/he stands fully erect and even less common that the back is bent backwards into extension.

In addition to the office worker we see evidence of this flexed posture in many other occupations such as the worker who stands throughout the day at a cash register or a workbench.

While Fahrni saw this flexed posture as a positive aspect it is reasonable to assume that other factors, such as increased flexibility and increased levels of fitness, may have contributed to the lower incidence of back pain that he saw in agrarian populations.

If we examine the stresses on the back during the day using the work of Nachemson et al. (5) we can see that the intervertebral disc is most vulnerable in the flexed, forward-bent position. This, it seems, is magnified in the seated position. It is no wonder that the patient presenting with back pain so often complains that s/he hurt the back while bending forward to pick up a pencil or reaching to lift a sack of groceries from the trunk of the car. It is worth noting at this point that, frequently, a worker injured on the job who is used to relatively heavy activities throughout the day is often allowed to return to work on some kind of "light duty" prior to a full release for his/her regular duties. This light duty often involves seated work for a few days with the assumption that this is easier on the recuperating individual. Serious consideration should be given whether to allow an injured worker, especially one in whom we suspect an intervertebral disc injury, to assume a seated position for any extended period of time. The evidence would seem to indicate that this may be counterproductive.

There are many examples of simple ergonomic modifications and lifestyle changes that have been used to minimize the stresses on our lower backs. By placing one foot on the bar rail in the local tavern the lumbar posture is altered sufficiently to allow the patron a more comfortable and relaxing time. This same concept, elevating one foot, has been used by counter workers, cashiers, assembly line workers, and many others. The use of the Balans chair, tilting table tops, etc. have also been used to enhance the natural curves of the lumbar spine.

In most discussions of posture we use the upright, erect position as the norm. Even the anatomy texts describe normal posture in this position. The problem that we face is most of us are rarely, if ever, in this so-called normal position. Janda (6) goes so far as to say that man is not a bipedal animal. Rather, he says, we usually stand on one leg at a time and he refers to man as a one-legged animal. He cites many examples of this single-legged stance and simple observation of a group of people waiting in line at the bank or at the grocery store is enough to convince us that Janda's observations are accurate.

Our posture continually changes throughout the day and we are faced with a never-ending array of demands on our musculoskeletal systems. Consequently, in our discussions of posture we must not be too hasty to refer to the "normal" upright posture found in the textbooks.

It seems that our posture is even influenced by our outlook on life. Consider the individual who is not feeling well or is depressed. S/he has a slumped, stooped posture and must continually respond to statements such as, "Are you feeling okay?" "You don't look like you feel well." Consider the opposite. The individual who is feeling particularly chipper and full of life. S/he walks erect, head up, shoulders back, chest out. It is not difficult to see that this person feels healthy.

2. IMPROPER DAILY HABITS

This area has received much of the attention in many programs that target back injury, particularly those in industry. One of the most often cited causes of lower back pain is improper daily habits, particularly lifting (7). Industry has spent a considerable amount of time and money to teach proper lifting procedures and this is one of the primary focuses of many industrial safety training programs.

It would appear that with so much effort directed at this single aspect, agreement would have been reached regarding the "best" way to lift. Not so. One group says that proper lifting involves keeping the back flat and reducing the lumbar lordosis (2) while a second group stresses the importance of arching or bowing the lower back in an effort to maintain the lumbar lordosis (8). However, both groups tend to agree on the following (Fig. 3.2):

a. Plant the feet firmly, placed slightly apart.
b. Bend the knees.

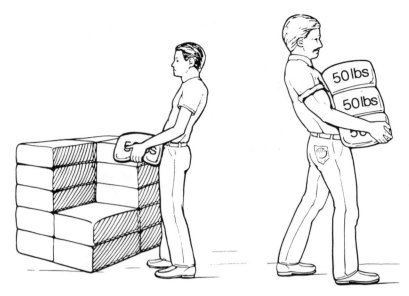

Figure 3.2. Proper lifting techniques are an important factor in preventing back injuries. (Adapted from Mayer T, Gatchel R: *Functional Restoration for Spinal Disorders: The Sports Medicine Approach.* Lea & Febiger, 1988.)

c. Keep the load close to the body.
d. Stay within personal limits.

Much of the effort in back injury prevention programs is focused around proper lifting techniques during the workday. It is important for the worker to understand that what s/he does off the job is equally important and that proper lifting does not just involve the workplace. Such routine duties as bending forward to pick up a dropped pencil or bending forward in the driveway to pick up the morning newspaper must be considered as potentially harmful and must be treated with the same attention as lifting a 90-pound sack of cement at the construction site.

As it is with so many other health problems, most people pay little attention to their back until it hurts. Only then do we give it any thought. We look for the slip, trip, object, or fall that caused the problem. One interesting study showed that compensated workers were better able to identify a specific incident with the onset of lower back pain. Kelsey (9) reported 70.9% of male workers receiving compensation associated lifting, falling, bending, carrying, pulling, or pushing with the onset of low back pain. Only 35.5% of the noncompensated workers made the same association. For female workers the respective percentages were 71.4 and 23.6. The evidence suggests that, in most instances, a single incidence of lifting is not the cause of back pain.

While teaching lifting techniques receives much of the attention, many other daily activities (collectively called activities of daily living or ADL) are implicated in the multifactorial causes of low back pain. These will be discussed in more detail in the "obstacle course."

3. POOR BODY MECHANICS

This component is perhaps the area that is least amenable to home care and is the area that often requires intervention by the chiropractor. The spine is a complex kinematic chain involving vertebrae, muscles, ligaments, nerves, etc. Proper functioning of this complex system is vital for the elimination of back pain and requires smooth coordinated interaction between all parts. Any single component that fails to function adequately will hamper the entire system and may contribute to its failure.

Perhaps one of the most important, and most frequently overlooked, links in this chain is the hip joint and the lumbar-pelvic rhythm. As we bend forward and backward movement occurs both at the hips and pelvis and in the lower portion of the lumbar spine. Any change or alteration in the functioning of the hip joint must be adapted to and may be seen in a compensatory hypermobility of the lumbar spine. It is my experience that proper evaluation and treatment of hypomobility of the acetabular joint can significantly reduce the stresses on the lumbar spine and relieve much discomfort.

Using this same rationale, it is possible to understand how dysfunction in any of the spinal joints may contribute to the development of lower back pain. Once again, I have seen many instances of back pain localized in the lower portion of the lumbar spine associated with hypomobility of the thoraco-lumbar junction, the thoracic spine, or the upper cervical spine. Restoration of normal function to these areas is often associated with significant relief of pain in the lower back.

It is important for the individual to recognize that early detection of functional deficiencies in this spinal kinematic chain may have a dramatic impact on the incidence of spinal degeneration. Kessler and Hertling (10) have stated that "subtle changes in the kinematics of synovial joints may lead to the development of osteoarthrosis." They continue by saying that "If we can detect and correct these small changes before gross pathology has developed, we may be able to delay, halt, or prevent the degenerative process itself." Gutmann and Wolff (11) stated that changes in function that were detectable by palpation and by dynamic radiographs would precede structural changes that could be detected by x-ray by a 10-year period.

Lewit (12) demonstrated in school-age children an alarming incidence of pelvic dysfunction. He found such pelvic distortion in 11 of 70 children between 14 and 41 months, in 81 of 181 between 3 and 6 years, and in 199 of 459 between 9 and 15 years. He stated that this pelvic dysfunction could be found in one-third to one-half of all children from nursery school on. He also found this was frequently associated with dysfunction in the upper cervical spine, particularly at the C0–C1 articulation. Lewit demonstrated that the pelvic dysfunction would often disappear upon manipulation of the upper cervical lesion (12).

In a separate study, Mieurau et al. (13) showed that 28.1% of children between the ages of 6 and 17 had identifiable pelvic dysfunction (sacroiliac joint hypomobility) and 23.5% had a history of back pain. It is reasonable to conclude that our efforts to prevent back pain should include evaluation of the function of the locomotor system of children as well as the adults who present with symptoms (14).

4. LOSS OF FLEXIBILITY

In addition to the flexed posture, our sedentary lifestyle has created an entire population that is extremely inflexible. In this author's opinion, there is an inverse relationship between the level of flexibility and the incidence of back pain and that perhaps one of the major contributing factors in the alarming incidence of back pain is decreasing flexibility. If we look at Fahrni's (1) early observations of ground-dwelling populations we can see that the crouched posture shown is associated with an increased flexibility of the entire spinal column.

Janda (14) has described a series of muscular changes that include a combination of weakened muscles and short, tight muscles. He has labeled these patterns the proximal and distal crossed syndromes. The pattern of muscular changes is as follows:

Muscles tending to shorten	Muscles tending to weaken
Upper body (upper crossed syndrome)	
Suboccipital	Neck flexors
Posterior cervicals	Rhomboids

Sternomastoid
Scalenes
Levator scapulae
Upper trapezius
Pectorals

Serratus anterior
Middle and lower trapezius

Lower body (lower crossed
    syndrome)
Erector spinae
Iliopsoas
Hamstrings
Piriformis
Tensor fasciae latae (TFL)
Quadratus lumborum
Gastrocnemius/soleus

Abdominals
Gluteals

Much of our effort directed at the muscles is aimed at strengthening the weakened muscles (i.e., abdominal curls, wall squats, etc.). More attention should be directed at the short, tight postural muscles. It has been shown that if we first take the time to stretch these short, tightened muscles such as the erector spinae, our efforts to strengthen the weak antagonist (abdominals) will be enhanced.

In a case study Janda described a woman with a long history of back pain who had failed to respond to many different treatment approaches. This 48-year-old woman demonstrated a typical pattern of weak abdominal muscles and tight trunk extensors. Strengthening exercises for the weak abdominals had been recommended but had made her condition worse. Electromyographic recordings demonstrated activity in the trunk extensors in all movements including movements in which they should be inactive. Thus, all exercises for strengthening the abdominals actually resulted in increased activity and strength of the trunk extensors. Stretching and inhibiting these trunk extensors had the effect of normalizing the interaction of the trunk flexors and extensors and improved the woman's condition substantially (14).

Janda (14) states that

It has been clinically proved that it is better to stretch the tight muscles first, thus inhibiting the weakened, inhibited antagonists. It is not exceptional that, after stretching of the tight muscle, the strength of the inhibited, weakened antagonist improves spontaneously, sometimes immediately, sometimes within a few days, without any additional treatment. By stretching it is sometimes possible to inhibit the tight muscle and to avoid undesirable overactivation during different movement patterns. This may be of great value in further exercise programmes.

With this in mind, much effort in the area of exercise protocols presented later in this text will be directed, not so much at strengthening weak muscles, but at stretching short, tight muscles. The reader is directed to Chapter 6 for specific information on this topic.

5. REDUCED LEVELS OF FITNESS

While the amount of money spent on health care in the United States is far greater than in any other country, it is generally accepted that the level of health of the average American is declining. This impacts all areas of the health care system, including the back pain patient. An encouraging trend in recent years had directed our attention at personal responsibility in prevention of health problems.

With regard to lower back pain, one study in 1979 by Cady et al. (15) compared the incidence of lower back pain in a group of Los Angeles firefighters. The firefighters in the study were grouped according to three levels of fitness, largely based on cardiovascular stamina, and followed for a period of 2 years during which the incidence of back injuries was recorded. Group 1 was termed "fit" and had an incidence of 1%. Group 2 was termed "moderately fit" and had a 3.5% incidence. Group 3 was termed "unfit" and had an 8% incidence of injury. This study concluded that there was a direct correlation between poor levels of fitness and back pain in workers performing the same tasks.

A significant component in reducing back pain should include efforts to improve aerobic fitness and to reduce other health risks such as obesity, smoking, blood pressure, etc. In an effort to gain some control over the rising cost of health care many industries have begun to regard the promotion of fitness in employees as one of their most important and promising weapons.

6. STRESS

Hans Selye (16) defined "disease" as "the bodies [sic] inability to cope with stress." Added to the factors previously described, the accumulating effects of a stress-filled lifestyle produce a "pro-inflammatory response" that magnifies the impact of otherwise moderate problems. Consequently, an important aspect of injury prevention is the reduction of stress and the use of relaxation therapy.

One application of relaxation therapy that I found particularly useful in private practice was the following. When a patient presented with an acute episode of low back pain it is sometimes difficult to properly evaluate the patient due to the extent of the pain and movement restriction. Either many of the tests cannot be performed because of the symptoms, or those that are performed are all positive anyway. Consequently, it may be difficult to determine the precise nature of the condition and to select the most appropriate treatment protocol. However, after I had completed my examination procedures including any necessary x-rays, I told the patient that it would take several minutes to develop the radiographs and that during this time I wanted them to relax. To help them accomplish this we placed the patient in a corner of the examination room on a therapy bench (see the "position of comfort" in Chapter 5). We provided an audio cassette with headphones and played a relaxation tape for the patient. The patient was then left for approximately 15–20 minutes during which time they were checked once or twice by a staff member. After relaxing in this position most patients felt some improvement and many fell asleep. It has been my observation that one of the first signs of improvement in a patient who has been in pain is a good night's sleep.

Kraus (17) cited tension and inadequate exercise as the two major cause of back pain. Mulry (18) claims the most dramatic and uniform effect of stress on the human body is an increase in physical tension. He states that when the individual, faced with increasing demands is unprepared or unable to adapt, it is predictable that muscles will tighten. It is not particularly important whether the demands are physical, emotional, or both; the reaction is the same. As the muscles tighten they increase pain, but the tightness also increases the likelihood of new or further injury to the tissue (18).

If we accept the premise that stress and tension are both a part of the cause of back pain and are amenable to treatment in the back pain patient then some method of assessing the level of stress must be used. To this end, Mulry (18) developed the Personal Concerns Inventory (PCI). This will be explained in Chapter 5.

References

1. Fahrni WH. *Backache and primal posture.* Vancouver: Musqueam Publishers, 1976.
2. Williams PC. *Low back and neck pain: causes and conservative treatment.* Springfield: Charles C. Thomas, 1974.

3. McKenzie R. *The lumbar spine, mechanical diagnosis and therapy.* Wellington, New Zealand: Spinal Publications, 1985.
4. Saunder HD. *Evaluation, treatment and prevention of musculoskeletal disorders.* Minneapolis: Viking Press, 1985:305–310.
5. Nachemson A, Morris J. In vivo measurements of intradiscal pressure. *J Bone Joint Surg* 1964;46A:1077–1092.
6. Janda MIV, personal communication, 1990.
7. Snook SH, Campanelli RA, Hart JW. A study of three preventive approaches to low back injury. *J Occup Med* 1978;20:478.
8. The American Back School, slide sound presentation.
9. Kelsey JL. An epidemiological survey of acute herniated lumbar intervertebral discs. *Rheumatol Rehabil* 1975;14:144–159.
10. Kessler RM, Hertling D. *Management of common musculoskeletal disorders.* Philadelphia: Harper and Row, 1983:11–49.
11. Gutmann G, Wolff HD. Die wirbelsaule als volkswirt-schaftlicher faktor. *Hippokrates* 1959;30:207.
12. Lewit K. *Manipulative therapy in rehabilitation of the locomotor system.* London: Butterworth, 1988:26–27.
13. Mieurau DR, Cassidy JD, Hamin T, Milne RA. Sacroiliac joint dysfunction and low back pain in school aged children. *J Manipulative Physiol Ther* 1984;7(2):81–84.
14. Janda MIV. Muscles, Motor regulation and back problems. In: Korr I, ed. *The neurobiologic mechanisms in manipulative therapy.* New York: Plenum Press, 1978:27–41.
15. Cady LD, Bischoff DP, O'Connell ER, et al. Strength and fitness and subsequent back injuries in firefighters. *J Occup Med* 1979;21:269.
16. Selye H. *Stress without distress.* Philadelphia: J.B. Lippincott, 1974.
17. Kraus H. *Backache, stress and tension.* New York: Simon and Schuster, 1965.
18. Mulry R. A functional psychological approach to low back pain. In: Brown F, ed. *Symposium on the lumbar spine.* St. Louis: C.V. Mosby, 1981:117–125.

4
Back Schools

The use of educational information to assist the back pain patient in avoiding future injuries is not new. Doctors have been counseling their patients in the proper ways of lifting, in exercise techniques, and in general health information for centuries. The use of the Back School as a formal method of providing patients with information is, however, relatively recent. The origin of the modern Back School can probably be traced to the work of W. H. Fahrni (1) in the late 1950s. Fahrni recognized the difference in occurrence of back pain between ground-dwelling populations and industrialized societies. He also realized that back pain, as a singular entity, is to some degree a controllable condition. Fahrni was one of the first doctors to train physical therapists to assist with the training of back pain patients.

The first reports of a formal Back School in the literature can be found in the early 1970s with the work of Zachrisson-Forsell (2). This was known as the Swedish Back School and was located in the Volvo factory. It was specifically designed for an industrial population and was, perhaps, a response by the consumer to a problem that the medical industry had failed to resolve (2,3).

The first statistical studies on the effectiveness of such procedures were published in the Scandinavian orthopedic journals in 1977 (4). At approximately the same time, Dr. Hamilton Hall in Toronto was developing a series of educational programs referred to as the Canadian Back Education Units (CBEU) (5). In San Francisco, Drs. Arthur White and Bill Matmiller were developing the California Back School (6). Since those early days some several thousand Back Schools have developed in the United States alone. Some are modeled after one of the early designs while others are structured around the individual philosophies and ideas of the developer.

41

Several of the Back School programs have been widely publicized and discussed and serve as a foundation for the "garden variety" back school that is found throughout the world. Of the more widely known, six have been reported in medical journals as being statistically effective; 1) the Australian program, 2) the Swedish Back School, 3) the Canadian Back Education Units (CBEU), 4) the California Back School, 5) the Fahrni method, and 6) the McKenzie method (7). While differing in individual emphasis and in philosophy of the developer, each of these methods consists of essentially the same type of information:

1. Back pain is a common occurrence.
2. There is no magic solution to the problem of back pain.
3. Information on low back anatomy and mechanics.
4. Information about the intervertebral disc and the aging process of the disc.
5. Posture and postural training.
6. Postural exercises.
7. Lifting techniques.
8. Body mechanics and movement training.
9. Exercises for strengthening pelvic, abdominal, and leg muscles.
10. Stretching exercises.

In addition, some Back School programs (California Back School, CBEU, etc.) also include information on the importance of stress management and relaxation techniques. All of these methods are designed with the same objectives in mind: to teach the patient how the back works, why problems develop, and to give them confidence to deal with painful situations, recurrent back pain, and difficult working conditions.

Statistics

Objective information regarding the efficacy of the Back School as a means of preventing back pain is not plentiful. Some studies have shown a significant improvement in overall patient condition with the education provided through the Back School (4,6,8,9). Other studies have shown that the Back School is no better, or no worse, than more common and more traditional treatment methods (10). That many other health problems such as polio and tuberculosis have been positively affected by patient education and prevention is indisputable, however. The general trend in health care toward more emphasis on education and prevention is consistent with the emergence of the Back School. In addition, the shift in attitude of the health care consumer (the patient) from one in which the doctor assumes the task of "healing" the patient to one in which the patient assumes primary responsibility for his/her own health has supported the growth of the Back School as an important component of caring for the back pain patient.

Dutro and Wheeler (11) claimed that research concerning Back School, although incomplete, is promising. They cite several studies that indicate that 85–97% of those attending Back Schools found the programs useful. In addition, 64–80% felt that the program had lowered their level of back pain. One of the most common aspects identified in such projects is the high level of patient satisfaction.

In addition to the studies cited, Dutro and Wheeler (11) claim that several examples from industry may be used to support the use of the Back School as part of a prevention program. Some examples are:

1. American Biltrite found a reduction in workers compensation claims of $180,000 to $40,000 at the end of a Back School program.
2. Southern Pacific Transportation Company (39,000 employees) instituted a back education program. The following year they saw a 22% decrease in the incidence of back injuries and a 43% decrease in lost work time. Their savings were calculated at $1,000,000 in a single year.
3. Clayton General Hospital in Georgia saw a drop in workers compensation costs from $118,000 to $27,000 in a single year. They attributed the reduction to a back school program.
4. Boeing Company utilized a back safety program with 3424 of its workers. 3500 other workers constituted a control group that had no such training. While the incidence of injury was similar for both groups there was some difference in lost work time; 4.2 days on average in those in the back school group versus 5.3 days in the control group.
5. PPG Industries used the Atlanta Back School program for 2000 of its workers. The injury rate in the subsequent 2 years was reduced by 70% and the costs by 90%.

Considering the enormous cost of health care and the large portion of that cost expended on workers with back injuries, these studies have tremendous significance.

One of the first studies cited in the literature was from Sweden by Berquist-Ullman and Larson in 1972 (4). They compared the response of 217 Volvo workers suffering from acute episodes of back pain. The workers were divided into three separate groups; 1) a back school only group, 2) a physical therapy group, and 3) a placebo group. The average duration of symptoms for the placebo group was 27.8 days while the duration for both the physical therapy group and the back school group was significantly less (15.9 and 14.8 days, respectively). The number of days off work was 26.5 for both the placebo group and the physical therapy group. The back school group missed, on average, 20.5 days. The recurrence of pain within the first year following the study was similar in all three groups. The authors concluded that when compared to the placebo group, both the back school and the physical therapy group had superior response in hastening recovery time. In addition they found that the back school was superior to both other groups in reducing lost work time (4).

In a separate study, Klaber-Moffett et al. (9) compared a back school approach with an exercise only group. As might be expected, both groups improved over a 6-week period. At 16 weeks, however, the exercise only group had reverted to their original pain levels whereas the back school subjects continued to show signs of improvement.

Hall and Iceton (8) have provided statistics for some 6418 individuals who participated in the CBEU. Subjects completed four lectures at weekly intervals with a follow-up review class held 6 months later. The average age of those in the study was 45.4 years with the ratio of men to women 4:6. The majority of the students were between the ages of 30 and 55. One significant difference between this study and that of Berquist-Ullman and Larson was the duration of symptoms. In the Hall and Iceton study more than 50% stated that they had back pain for longer than 3 years. A single attack was reported by only 6% while 40% reported intermittent acute episodes with pain-free periods in between. A full 31% reported continuous pain with superimposed attacks and 23% reported continuous daily pain with no recurrent acute attacks. At the beginning of the lecture series 44% of the patients stated that their pain was stable, 29% felt that their condition was improving, while 27% felt that it was deteriorating. When questioned at the review class, 64% felt that their back pain had improved. Only 6.4% felt that their condition was worsening while 25.8% reported no pain at all. 97% stated that the program had helped (8).

A review of the first 300 patients of the California Back School found that 89% had not sought further medical treatment during 9 months following the back school. Ninety-five percent were able to resume normal activities after 1 month and were successful at retaining these activities during a 2-year follow-up period (6).

It is difficult to compare the results of different back school studies without knowing the particular aspects of the individual patients participating in the program. The study by Berquist-Ullman and Larson involved mainly acute back pain patients from a single industrial setting. That of Hall and Iceton involved a variety of chronic back pain patients from many segments of society, patients who had not responded to other types of care. The response of the individual who is involved in some type of litigation or "secondary gain" is know to be poorer than the individual who is not compensated. The effectiveness of the program design itself, or the nature of the instructors, is also an issue that is difficult to gauge.

With all of the problems involved in developing adequate comparative statistics, one thing seems clear; patient attitude is positively affected by attempts to teach them about their back and their condition. All of the studies cited indicate a high level of patient satisfaction with the information gained and the time spent. The underlying premise of back schools is that those patients who understand their conditions will fare better than those who do not.

BACK SCHOOL PROGRAMS
The Swedish Back School (12)

This consists of four lessons that are accomplished over a 2-week period. Each lesson lasts approximately 45 min and includes a 15-min sound-slide presentation followed by a 30-min presentation by a physical therapist. The class consists of 6–8 subjects. The goals of the Swedish program are: 1) to create self-confidence so that patients may manage their own back conditions, 2) to avoid potentially harmful treatment through better patient understanding of the role treatment plays in their condition, and 3) to reduce the escalating cost of medical care for low back patients.

The first class concentrates on the anatomy and mechanics of the back, the development of back pain, and the types of treatment methods used. Resting positions are taught and some treatment advice is given.

The second lesson focuses on the stresses on the back that develop from poor posture and the improper performance of manual tasks such as lifting, etc. Attention is directed at exercising the abdominal muscles in an effort to strengthen them.

The third lesson involves a practical application of information derived during the first two lessons. Activities of daily living are illustrated and practiced and the patient is taught how to get in and out of bed, out of chairs, etc.

The fourth class stresses the need for physical activity and reviews the information from the first three sessions. The patient is provided with a written summary prior to being dismissed.

The Canadian Back Education Units (CBEU) (5)

This program consists of four 90-min lectures that are held at weekly intervals. Each class consists of 15–20 individuals. The first lesson deals with anatomy, mechanics, and the aging process of the spine and is taught by an orthopedic surgeon. The second class, taught by a physical therapist, concentrates on proper body mechanics and on methods used for obtaining temporary relief from back pain. Class three is taught by a psychiatrist and deals with the psychiatric aspects of chronic pain and the influence of emotions on back pain. The final class is taught by a psychologist and a physical therapist together. The psychologist demonstrates relaxation exercises and the physical therapist teaches some basic exercise techniques (flexion exercises, isometric exercises, and pelvic tilt). A pre-test, a test at the end of the lectures, and a final test of the review class are used.

As part of the CBEU, patients are scheduled for a review class that takes place approximately 6 months after completion of class four. In their review article, Hall and Iceton stated that only 38% of 6418 patients who attended the original course return for the 6-month review. This is similar to this author's experience.

The California Back School (13)

The California Back School is somewhat different and more intensive and includes three 90-min sessions held at weekly intervals with a follow-up visit 1 month later. Class size is small, consisting of four patients in each group. Much of the class is taught by a physical therapist using a sound-slide program to provide information on the anatomy and mechanics of the back.

The first class includes basic information on the natural history of back pain, activities that aggravate back pain, and on the anatomy and aging of the spine. In addition, information on how pain can be relieved and activities of daily living is provided. One of the unique features of this program involves the methods used to evaluate the patient. An obstacle course is incorporated to objectively rate individual performance, along with an exercise tolerance test.

The second class concentrates on activities of daily living (ADL), on coordination exercises and on training at the obstacle course. Participants are taught a program of exercises and back safety on the job.

The third class includes a quiz on the information provided thus far, along with a final test on the obstacle course. Instruction is given on handling different size and shape loads and on safe back habits for sports and recreation. The patient is provided with a Personal Concerns Inventory (PCI) and instructed on its use. They are to return the completed PCI at the next visit.

The final class follows 1 month after class three. It is primarily a problem-solving day during which the patient is again tested on the obstacle course. In addition, the PCI is reviewed and suggestions made regarding ways of modifying individual problem areas.

Of the three back school programs discussed, the Swedish Back School is the most general and, as such, is useful to patients with acute and/or chronic back pain. The CBEU is designed more to deal with chronic back pain and attempts to change the patients' attitudes about the problem. The California Back School attempts to individualize the program to the specific needs of the patient and incorporates the program in the diagnosis and treatment aspects. One important aspect of the California Back School is its emphasis on stress management and relaxation.

Each of the Back School programs here described has value and may serve as a useful outline for the development of such a program in the chiropractic practice. Most individuals will find that, while the general format is satisfactory, some modifications are helpful to properly adapt the Back School to the individual needs and personalities of the practitioner. In the following chapter we will provide some useful suggestions that may easily be incorporated as your program is developed.

References

1. Fahrni WH. *Backache and primal posture.* Vancouver: Musqueam Publishers, 1976.
2. Zachrisson M. *The low back school.* Danderyd, Sweden: Danderyd's Hospital sound and slide program, 1972.
3. Zachrisson-Forsell M. The Swedish back school. *Physiotherapy* April 1980;66.
4. Berquist-Ullman M, Larson U. Acute low back pain in industry. *Acta Orthop Scan* Suppl 1977;170.
5. Hall H. The Canadian back education units. *Physiotherapy* 1980;66(4):118.

6. Matmiller AW. The California back school. *Physiotherapy* 1980;66(4):115.

7. Fisk JR, DiMonte P, McKay Courington S. Back Schools, Past, Present and Future. *Clin Orthop* October 1983;179:18–23.

8. Hall H, Iceton JA. Back school: An overview with specific reference to the Canadian back education units. *Clin Orthop* October, 1983;179:10–17.

9. Klaber-Moffett JA, Chase SM, Portek I, Ennis JR. A controlled perspective study to evaluate the effectiveness of a back school in the relief of chronic low back pain. *Spine* 1986;11:120–122.

10. Kvien TK, Nilsen H, Vik P. Education and self-care of patients with low back pain. *Scand J Rheumatol* 1981;10:318–320.

11. Dutro CL, Wheeler L. Back school and chiropractic practice. *J Manipulative Physiol Ther* September, 1986;9:209–212.

12. Zachrisson-Forsell M. The Back School. *Spine* January, 1981;6:104–106.

13. White AH. *Back school and other conservative approaches to low back pain.* St. Louis: C.V. Mosby, 1983.

5

Implementation of a Back School Program into Chiropractic Practice

During the 20 years since 1969 many different back schools have developed. Various estimates place the number of formal back schools in the United States at over 2000. While the basic purpose, the goals and the information supplied remain similar from one program to the next there is a wide variety in the manner in which the information is presented, the emphasis on particular aspects of the program, the number of sessions, the number of individuals in a class, the training of the instructors, and the amount of follow-up. The purpose of this chapter is to provide the reader with several different viable options that will facilitate the implementation of a Back School into the chiropractic practice.

Before proceeding it should be appreciated that the requirements and demands of your particular situation must be taken into account. Many well-meaning individuals have attempted to establish some type of ongoing patient education program only to find that the logistics were complicated and impractical. As with any patient education program, the Back School will change as your time, energy, and experience change. With this in mind, we will take a look at what it takes to implement a Back School.

As stated in Chapter 4, the first Back School consisted of four separate sessions given over a 2-week period. Each session had six to eight participants and was led by a physiotherapist. A slide-sound program was incorporated to facilitate the teaching and to ensure that all of the information was covered. While this format has been adopted in general by many it is not practical for each instance.

To determine the optimum Back School program that is both effective and practical the following should be considered:

a. Patient population
b. Available space
c. Personnel
d. Available time
e. Available equipment
f. Fees

Patient Population

One of the primary considerations in developing a Back School is the nature of the intended participants and the demographics of the community in which the school will function. Those participating in a Back School may be current back pain patients, a general patient population, worker's compensation back injuries, participants in an industrial safety program, school-age children, lay groups, and many others. The particular design of your Back School must take into account the variable characteristics of the population that it is intended to reach. In many instances, it may be necessary or helpful to develop several different formats aimed at reaching different groups.

For example, if your primary focus is an industrial population, large group settings with a couple of class sessions are more readily accomplished than one-on-one training that extends over a prolonged time period. There may be certain individuals in a given industry, however, who have a chronic and complicated history of back problems who would benefit more from an individualized program. Likewise, if you are lecturing to a lay group as part of a community service, you will find a large group setting to be most productive. Once again, those individuals in the group who have a history of problems may choose a more directed and individualized program.

Available Space

Do you have separate facilities that will be dedicated to patient education or are you going to "double up" with a space that is used for other activities? If space is a problem small groups or even one-on-one programs will be more practical. You may also have to consider scheduling Back School sessions at a time when the office is not involved in patient treatment activities.

If your Back School is to include an obstacle course and an exercise area, and space is not a problem, you will need an open room with approximately 200 square feet of floor space. The only requirements are that the room be carpeted and clean.

If you choose to have a Back School that consists of a large group lecture format and space is a problem you may want to consider renting a small meeting room in a local hotel. You should also inquire at the local public library, a nearby public school, church, or perhaps a fitness center as many have rooms that will suit your needs.

Personnel

One of the most important questions that should be asked is, Who is going to instruct in your Back School? Are you going to provide the instruction yourself? Are you going to use existing personnel or are you going to add an additional individual specifically for this purpose? If you hire someone, who is going to train him/her?

Saunders (1) states that "only those people who are well qualified and who are good teachers . . . will have significant success in this area." By this he means a physical therapist or some other individual who has received specific training. However, a great deal can often be accomplished with existing office staff. In my experience it is always better to select an individual who has had a history of back pain. S/he needs to be friendly, uninhibited, and willing to listen and learn. In every community there are people with some health and/or education experience (PTs, LPNs, RNs, retired teachers, etc.) who are eager and willing to work a few hours a day and enjoy interacting with people. An ad in a local newspaper should provide a list of qualified people. You may even find the right person in your patient files. (Note: this should not be viewed as an opportunity to recruit new patients. Be serious about finding the right person for the job and your Back School will have a much better chance of succeeding).

Whoever you employ for this purpose, somebody has to train him/her. There are many resources available to facilitate this and you are encouraged to take advantage of them.

Available Time

Are you planning to schedule Back School sessions during the normal work day while patient care is being administered? If so, you will need both space and personnel dedicated solely to this purpose. Or are you willing to schedule Back School sessions during non-peak office hours, during evenings, or on weekends? Remember, you may have to begin with a "less-than-ideal" arrangement to get things started.

Available Equipment

What are your equipment needs? One of the distinct advantages of a Back School is that you will not need a great deal of sophisticated or expensive equipment. Most of the time you will be using things found around the house such as a vacuum cleaner, suitcase, floor mop, grocery sacks, etc. You will find it helpful, however, to have either a slide projector, cassette tape recorder, and/or a television with a video cassette recorder.

Fees

Perhaps one of the most practical questions is how much should you charge and who is to pay? Fees vary from location to location but a reasonable fee is the cost of an extended office visit. Many insurance companies will pay for these services and you may find the patient's employer willing to pay. Whatever the cost, and whoever pays the bill, it has been stated that, for every one dollar spent on education and prevention, nine dollars are saved.

Taking the Plunge

As you plan your Back School consider the options that are most practical for your situation and begin. Appreciate that you will undoubtedly make changes as you gain experience. There are many questions that will remain unanswered and you may be uncertain about the chances of success. If you wait until you have all of your questions answered and you have secured the best possible facility, staff, and format chances are you will never start. One thing is certain, the chances of your Back School succeeding are much better once you begin.

BACK SCHOOL VARIATIONS

In the following section I have described a variety of different options. Regardless of the format the following topics should be covered:

a. Anatomy
b. Body mechanics
c. Posture
d. First aid
e. Exercise
f. Stress reduction
g. General health and fitness

Large Groups (25–30 Participants)

While this is not the most effective format for teaching a Back School it does offer many distinct advantages that make it a practical and cost-effective method. It is also very adaptable for safety presentations in an industrial setting or as a public service to community groups. In addition, this may be a good way of introducing yourself, your staff, and your patients to the Back School concepts. It must be remembered that the purpose of the Back School is to provide information in a useable manner in an effort to reduce the frequency of back injury. This should *not* be considered a "lay lecture" nor should it be used to "sell" patients on the virtues of chiropractic care.

A formal lecture or classroom setting with an instructor and an occasional audio-visual presentation is considered a "passive learning" situation and is not a very effective way of educating. The participants need to be somehow "actively" involved in the learning process and not just talked to.

Rather than a classroom setting with rows of desks it is suggested that you use an open, carpeted space approximately 200 square feet equipped simply with folding chairs and large pillows. Begin with the chairs arranged in a circle around the perimeter of the room.

Each participant is expected to attend two sessions that are spaced no further apart than 7–10 days. They should be told in advance that they will be expected to actively participate and should dress comfortably in loose fitting clothing such as "sweats." Each participant should be asked to bring two pillows.

Session One

Begin the first session by introducing yourself as a fellow back pain patient (since 80% of the population is said to have back pain at some point in their lifetime it is safe to assume that you are). Ask how many are currently having pain and caution them that they are to inform you if they develop difficulty during either of the sessions.

Briefly outline the purpose of the Back School: 1. Self-care and rehabilitation; 2. Alteration in body mechanics; 3. Prevention of recurring pain.

It should be emphasized at this point that (*a*) back pain is only a symptom that represents a loss of health and is not the result of a single incident, and (*b*) there is *no* magic cure for back pain.

The single most important aspect of the Back School is to get the individual to accept the responsibility for his/her own back.

While the participants are seated it is helpful to consider some of the statistics relevant to the back pain problem. Most people, particularly those with chronic pain, are somewhat reassured to find that they are not alone.

This introduction should be kept relatively short, preferably less than 10 minutes. At this point ask the group the following questions:

A. What causes back pain?
   1. Poor posture
   2. Poor daily living habits (lifting, etc.)
   3. Poor body mechanics
   4. Loss of flexibility
   5. Reduced levels of fitness
   6. Stress
B. What were you doing the first time that you hurt your back? The last time?
C. How did you react the last time you hurt your back?
   1. Fear
   2. Irritation
   3. Anger
   4. Stress
D. Do you think this reaction helped your condition or hurt it?
E. What should you do if you hurt your back again?
   RELAX.

One of the most important aspects of back injury prevention is minimizing the consequences of future episodes. Regardless of how knowledgeable an individual may be, accidents happen and we make mistakes. We can assume that future back problems will probably occur. But, the reaction of the patient at the time will have a significant impact on the seriousness of the episode. The purpose of this portion of the Back School is to teach relaxation in "the position of comfort" (2).

Ask the group to remember the most comfortable position they could find during their last attack. Usually it is flat on their back with knees bent (the semi-Fowler's position). At this point, ask the group to place their pillows on the floor and lay in this position with one pillow under the head and the other under the knees. From this point on everyone should refer to this position as the "position of comfort" (Fig. 5.1). (Be sure to point out that if anyone is not comfortable they should move into a more comfortable position at this time.)

The group should be informed that this position is helpful in reducing the pressure in the intervertebral disc and has a significant therapeutic effect.

The next portion involves using a relaxation tape, either audio cassette or video tape. Explain to the participants that they should listen to the tape and follow the instructions. Dim the lights in the room and begin the tape. Allow approximately 10 min for this relaxation exercise. I have always enjoyed this portion of the program the most and am always pleased with the distinct change in the reactions of the group following the relaxation phase.

Once the time is up ask the group to roll onto their side and gradually come back to reality. Only then should they sit up and return to their chair. Participants should be encouraged to repeat this procedure daily and should set aside a time for relaxation. It should be stressed that this is one of the most helpful aspects of the

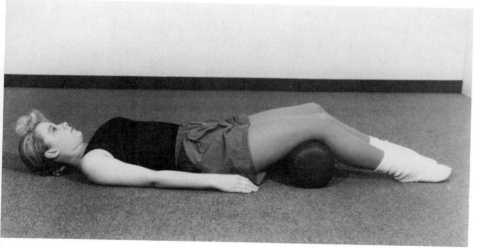

Figure 5.1. Relax in "the position of comfort."

Back School program and benefits their general health and well-being. It is helpful if you are able to provide participants with an audio cassette for their home use.

At this point a brief overview of the anatomy and function of the spine is helpful. This is an area of many Back Schools that often becomes too elaborate. While it has been shown that patient satisfaction improves with their level of understanding of the function of their back, most people will not remember complex anatomical concepts and terms. Therefore, keep it simple. It is suggested that you allow no more than 10 minutes for this description.

The next step involves teaching some elementary lifting skills. While there are several different views regarding the most effective techniques, each has several features in common. Rather than stressing details it is important to have the group experience the proper lifting procedure.

Pick someone from the group who looks fairly athletic and ask him/her to come to the middle of the room. You are going to have a "tug-of-war" with him/her that will demonstrate the wrong lifting mechanics. Ask your volunteer to stand with feet together, knees locked, and arms outstretched. Have him/her hold onto the rope and when ready resist your efforts to pull him/her over. In this position s/he is not very strong and is easily pulled off balance.

Now ask your helper to position him/herself so that s/he can win the tug-of-war. With rare exceptions s/he will spread the feet, bend the knees, hold the stomach in, and grasp the rope close to the body. This is a powerful position that Mulry calls "the position of strength" and is the preferred lifting posture (Fig. 5.2).

To demonstrate the importance of each component, ask the group to stand and pair up facing each other. Have one member of each pair stand with feet together, knees locked and arms outstretched. Instruct the individual to avoid using any abdominal muscles while the partner attempts to lower his/her arms.

Next, ask the participants to assume the position of strength and resist attempts to further lower the arms. They should immediately experience a significant increase in strength and stability. Change partners and repeat the exercise. This demonstration is graphic and serves to reinforce the concept of: (a) feet apart, (b) knees bent, (c) tighten abdomen, and (d) keep the load close.

The group should be encouraged to remember this "position of strength" when lifting any object, regardless of its size.

The final phase of this first class is stress reduction. A brief description of stress and the impact on the musculoskeletal system

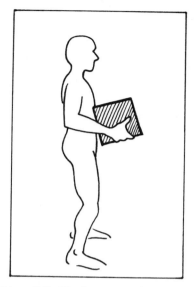

Figure 5.2. The "position of strength."

is suggested. Ask the group to describe how they feel when they are stressed: (a) uptight, (b) a bundle of nerves, or (c) tied in knots.

It is no coincidence that stress is described in such somatic terms.

Distribute a copy of the Personal Concerns Inventory (Fig. 5.3) and describe its use. Each individual is to check the areas that are particularly stressful on a daily basis and indicate on a scale of 1 to 10 the degree to which they are a problem. They should bring the PCI to the next session.

Answer any questions that the group might have. Thank them for their attention and assistance and reinforce the following:

a. Back pain is not the result of a single incident.
b. There is no magic solution to the back pain problem.
c. Their back is *their* responsibility.

Remind the group of the next meeting time and dismiss them.

Session Two

The topics to be discussed in this second session are: (a) relaxation, (b) proper body mechanics, (c) exercises and flexibility, and (d) stress reduction.

	DAY 1	DAY 2	DAY 3	DAY 4	DAY 5	DAY 6	DAY 7	TOTAL	DAY 1	DAY 2
Need More Recreation										
Noise at Home										
Noise at Work										
Sleeping Problems										
Chest Pain										
Problems with Children										
Weight Problems										
Need to be more Assertive										
Recent Death in Family										
High Blood Pressure										
Conflicts with Relatives										
Poor Eating Habits										
Short Temper										
Freeway Traffic										
Cigarette Smoking										
Feel Guilty										
Back Pain										
Alcohol (self)										
Alcohol (other)										
Jealousy										
Pill Consumption										
Boredom										
Tension										
Worry Too Much										
Medical Bills										
Need Employment										
Divorce										
Separation										
Dislike Job										
Continued Physical Pain										
Job Security										
Unexpressed Anger										
Headaches										
Trouble Making Decisions										
Conflicts With Neighbors										
Marital Problems										
Financial Difficulties										
Desire More Social Life										
Need to Relax										
Trouble with Employer										
Need Physical Exercise										
Need Friends										
Nervousness										
Sex Difficulties										
More Time for Myself										
Deadlines on Job										
Depression										
Can't Say No										
Ulcers										
Loneliness										
General Unhappiness										
More Self Discipline										
TOTAL										

Figure 5.3. The Personal Concerns Inventory. (Adapted from White AH. *Back school and other conservative approaches to low back pain.* St. Louis: C.V. Mosby, 1983.

Begin the session with a quick review of the first class. Ask for any questions or concerns. Have the group assume the position of comfort and start the relaxation tape (allow 10 min). Once the tape is over arouse the group slowly as you did before and ask them to return to their chairs.

Have two or three people come to the center of the room and drop several one dollar bills on the floor. Ask each to pick up one of the bills. If they bend at the knees instead of the waist let them keep the money.

Have someone else come to the center of the room and lift a heavier object such as a suitcase or a grocery sack. You may repeat this with different size and different weight objects. Remind the group of the components of the position of strength.

The next step is to assess the flexibility of each individual. Have the group pair up and complete the flexibility and strength tests included (Fig. 5.4).

After performing the tests for flexibility and strength, demonstrate the suggested exercises and have the group perform each one. It is important to point out that they should stretch but not strain and should stop if they have any pain. A little soreness, however, is usually a good sign.

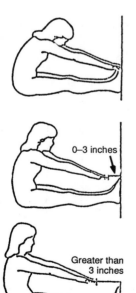

1. Back bending flexibility

   Purpose: to test the flexibility of the hamstrings and the low back muscles.

   Method: sit on the floor, feet flat against the wall, legs extended and straight. Touch the tips of your toes with your fingertips.

   Scoring: if you can extend your fingertips to the tips of your toes — GOOD.

   If you can extend your fingertips to within 3 inches of your toes — MARGINAL.

   If you are unable to extend your fingertips to within 3 inches of your toes —UNSATISFACTORY.

Figure 5.4. Back screening tests assessing strength and flexibility. (Courtesy of Back Care Center, Leawood, Kansas.)

2. Abdominal strength:

   Purpose: to test the strength of the abdominal muscles.

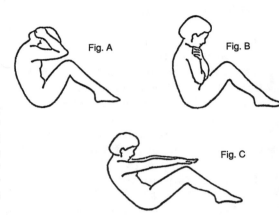

   Method: lie on your back on the floor. Place your hands behind your head and sit up. Next, place your hands across your chest, then extend your arms toward your knees and sit up.

   Scoring: if you can sit up like figures A and B — GOOD. If only like figure C — MARGINAL. If you are unable to do a sit-up — UNSATISFACTORY.

3. Unilateral hamstring stretch:

   Purpose: to test the flexibility of the hamstring muscles

   Method: lie on the floor on your back with your legs straight. Raise one leg as far as you can, keeping the knee straight. Repeat with the other leg.

   Scoring: if you are able to raise to 80° or more — GOOD

   If you are able to raise to 60–80° — MARGINAL

   If you are unable to raise your legs to 60° — UNSATISFACTORY

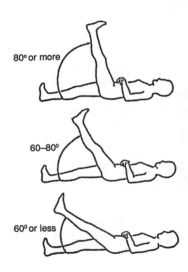

Figure 5.4. *Continued.*

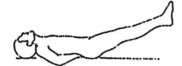

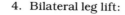

4. Bilateral leg lift:

Purpose: to test the strength of the abdominal muscles, hip flexors, and knee extensor muscles.

Method: lie on your back on the floor with your knees straight and your legs extended. Lift both legs to 15 inches off the floor and hold this position.

Scoring: if you are able to maintain this position for 10 seconds or more — GOOD

If you can assume the position, but are unable to maintain it — MARGINAL

If you are unable to assume the position — UNSATISFACTORY

5. Back extension flexibility:

Purpose: to test the ability of the back to extend

Method: lie on your stomach on the floor with your arms directly under your shoulders. Lift your body with your arms, keeping the iliac crest on the floor.

Scoring: if the iliac crest is either flush with the floor or within 2 inches of the floor — GOOD

If the iliac crest is 2–4 inches from the floor — MARGINAL

If the iliac crest is 4 or more inches from the floor — UNSATISFACTORY

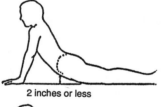

2 inches or less

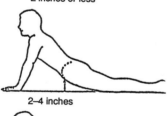

2–4 inches

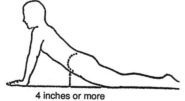

4 inches or more

Figure 5.4. *Continued.*

6. Back strength:

Purpose: to test the overall strength of the back muscles

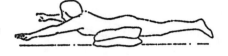

Method: lie on the floor with your arms and legs extended. Place 2 pillows under your pelvis. Lift your chest and legs off the floor.

Scoring: if you are able to maintain this position for 10 seconds or more — GOOD

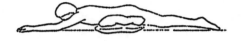

If you can assume the position, but are unable to maintain it —MARGINAL

If you are unable to assume the position — UNSATISFACTORY

Figure 5.4. *Continued.*

Note: perhaps the major disadvantage of such a large group is the impracticality of developing an individual exercise program. Consequently, the exercises given have been selected because they are considered both safe and helpful.

Exercises (Figs. 5.5–5.22):
a. Knee-to-chest (supine and/or side-lying).
b. Pelvic tilt (supine or standing).
c. Low back extensor stretching (on hands and knees).
d. Low back extensor stretching (supine).
e. Low back extensor stretching (sitting).
f. Hip abductor strengthening (side-lying).
g. Hip extensor strengthening (prone).
h. Hip extensor strengthening (supine).
i. Hamstring stretching (sitting).
j. Hamstring stretching (supine).
k. Hip flexor stretching (supine).
l. Hip flexor stretching (side-lying).
m. Abdominal strengthening (supine).
n. Tensor fasciae latae (TFL) stretching (supine).

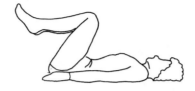

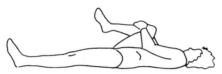

Figure 5.5. Knee-to-chest exercise (supine and/or side-lying). (Figures 5.5–5.22 are adapted from LaFreniere JG. *The low back patient.* New York: Masson Publishing, USA, 1979.)

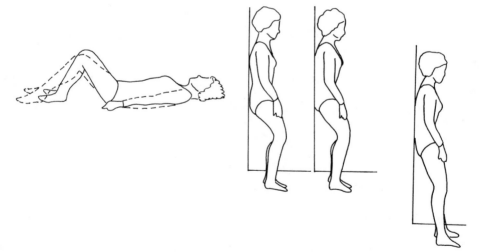

Figure 5.6. Pelvic tilt exercise (supine or standing).

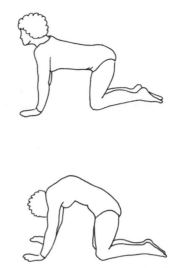

Figure 5.7. Low back extensor stretching (on hands and knees).

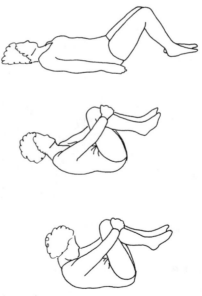

Figure 5.8. Low back extensor stretching (supine).

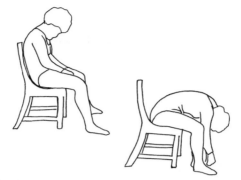

Figure 5.9. Low back extensor stretching (sitting).

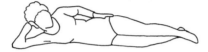

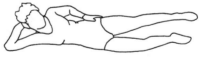

Figure 5.10. Hip abductor strengthening (side-lying).

o. TFL stretching (seated).
p. TFL stretching (side-lying).
q. Hip adductor stretching (supine).
r. Hip adductor stretching (sitting).

After practicing each of the exercises the group should be encouraged to set aside some time each day for relaxation and for exercises, especially the flexibility exercises. They should be encouraged to call if problems are encountered or questions arise.

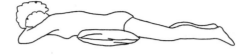

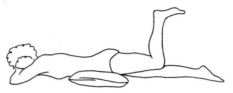

Figure 5.11. Hip extensor strengthening (prone).

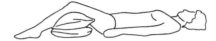

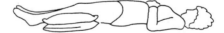

Figure 5.12. Hip extensor strengthening (supine).

The final step in this session is to review the Personal Concerns Inventory (PCI). Each participant should review those problem areas that are indicated. It is often more effective to pass the PCIs around the room and ask for suggestions regarding solutions.

After completing the review of the PCI you should field any questions. Finally, prior to dismissing the class, encourage them to continue with what they have learned and wish them well.

Small Group Sessions (6–8 Participants)

This is perhaps one of the most common formats for Back School presentations and is similar to the one used in the original Back

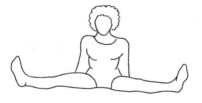

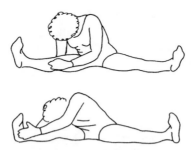

Figure 5.13. Hamstring stretching (sitting).

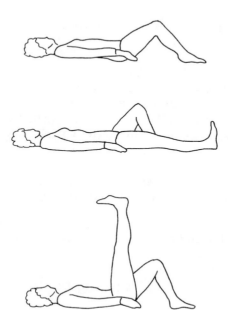

Figure 5.14. Hamstring stretching (supine).

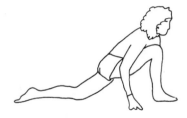

Figure 5.15. Hip flexor stretching (supine).

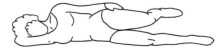

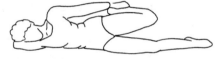

Figure 5.16. Hip flexor stretching (side-lying).

School of Zachrisson-Forsell. There are some distinct advantages to this format and class size, particularly the amount of individual attention that may be given. Because of this, more time can be devoted to developing individual exercise programs and resolving individual work-related and daily activity problems.

Session One

It is suggested that the first session be identical to that described for large groups. The topics to be covered are:

a. Introduction
b. The causes of back pain
c. What to do if you hurt your back
d. The position of comfort
e. Relaxation

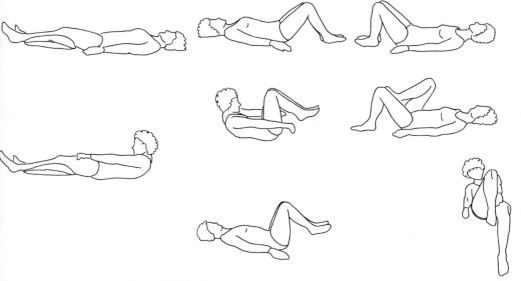

Figure 5.17. Abdominal strengthening (supine).

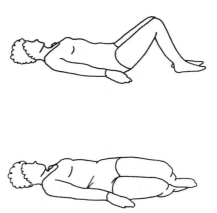

Figure 5.18. TFL stretching (supine).

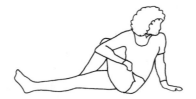

Figure 5.19. TFL stretching (seated).

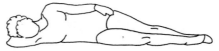

Figure 5.20. TFL stretching (side-lying).

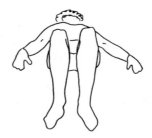

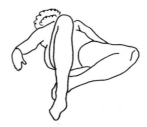

Figure 5.21. Hip adductor stretching (supine).

Session Two

The topics to be discussed in this second session will include:

a. Review
b. Relaxation
c. Lifting

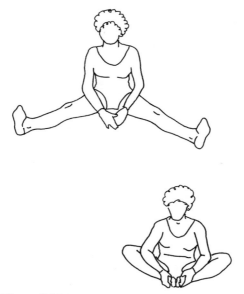

Figure 5.22. Hip adductor stretching (sitting).

d. Obstacle course
e. Exercises and flexibility
f. Stress

Begin session two in the same manner as before with a review of the first class and a relaxation period. Once again, encourage the participants to develop a daily habit of this exercise.

The next topic to address is the lifting skills. Begin this, as before, by placing several one dollar bills on the floor and asking each individual to pick one up. Those using correct procedures are allowed to keep the bills.

Obstacle Course

With this smaller group it is suggested that you incorporate some form of obstacle course in the second session. The obstacle course consists of a series of common activities of daily living that each participant must perform. Each is scored based on observation of performance as shown in the score sheet (Fig. 5.23).

The obstacle course will require additional equipment. Select any and/or all of the following:

GENERAL OBSTACLE COURSE

PATIENT NAME _____

ACTIVITY:	SCORE	POINTS	SCORE
Sitting, Relaxed:			
Low back support		2 2	
No kyphosis		1 1	
Semi-reclining position		1 1	
Knees at or higher than hips		1 1	
Sitting, Work-intensive Position:			
Low back support		1 1	
No kyphosis		2 2	
Knee clearance		1 1	
Standing, Relaxed:			
Minimal lordosis		1 1	
Minimal kyphosis		1 1	
Head centered		1 1	
Knees slightly flexed		1 1	
Walking:			
Minimal lordosis		1 1	
Minimal kyphosis		1 1	
No limp		1 1	
Feet apart		1 1	
Reaching:			
Minimal lordosis — pelvic tilt		2 2	
Knees slightly flexed		1 1	
Bending:			
Knee flexion greater than spine flexion		1 1	
Spine straight — shoulders retracted		1 1	
Pelvic tilt upon arising		2 2	
Kneeling or Crouching:			
One knee on floor		1 1	
Shoulders retracted		1 1	

Figure 5.23. Obstacle course. (Adapted from White AH. *Back school and other conservative approaches to low back pain.* St. Louis: C.V. Mosby, 1983.

Lifting:

Knee flexion greater than spine flexion	1	1
Pelvic tilt upon lifting	2	2
Load held close to body	1	1
Spine straight — shoulders retracted	1	1
Feet wide apart	1	1

Twisting:

Minimal lordosis — Pelvic tilt	2	2
Pivot motion as one unit	1	1

Side Bending:

Knee flexion greater than spine flexion	1	1
Pelvic tilt upon arising	2	2

Pushing and Pulling:

Knees flexed	1	1
Pelvic tilt	1	1

Over and Under:

Over: Minimal lordosis — Pelvic tilt	1	1
Under: Spine straight — Shoulders retracted	1	1
Pelvic tilt upon arising	2	2

Resting Positions:
Lying on the back:

Head upon moderate pillow	1	1
Knees flexed	1	1

Side-lying:

Head upon moderate pillow	1	1
Knees drawn up — "C" position	1	1

Lying on the abdomen:

No head pillow or elevation	1	1
Pillow under abdomen	1	1

TOTAL	_____	50 50	_____
Percent score	_____ %		_____ %

COMMENTS:

Figure 5.23. *Continued.*

Suitcase weighing approximately 15 pounds
Grocery sack with weights
A 20-pound sack of dog food
Vacuum cleaner
Lawnmower
Ironing board
Garden rake
Shelves at different heights
Doll in a car seat
Grocery cart
A 5-gallon bottle of water
Snowshovel
Auto tire

Be creative and add to this list anything that you find helpful.

Have the group divide into pairs and select five or six different tasks for the obstacle course for each pair. If you allow the participants to score each other you will be free to pass around the room and lend assistance and/or answer questions. (You might also find it helpful to videotape the activities and play them back to the group when they are finished. We have found this to be a most helpful tool.)

Allow approximately 15–20 minutes for the obstacle course. Assemble in a classroom setting and review the scores for the obstacle course. The group should, at this point, be aware of their own weaknesses and areas of concern. Answer any questions regarding the activities performed and ask the group to bring any different activities not covered to the third session.

The final portion of this class is the PCI. Spend a few minutes discussing problem areas and encourage participants to use the relaxation skills they are developing on a daily basis.

Session Three

The focus of the third session will be on exercise. As stated earlier, one of the primary advantages of small group sessions is the ability to work with each participant individually. The particular needs of each person can be addressed and an exercise program tailored to them.

Begin the session as before with a relaxation period. This is a most important step and has many benefits. In addition to the physical relaxation it tends to focus the individual's attention to the task at hand. Do not skip the relaxation step.

A brief description of the purpose and types of exercises is helpful at this point. For our purposes, we categorize the exercises into the following groups:

a. Exercises for flexibility and mobility;
b. Exercises for strength and endurance;
c. Exercises for cardiovascular fitness (aerobic);
d. Exercises for balance and coordination.

The first step is to assess the flexibility and strength of the group using the format described previously (Session Two — large group setting).

Flexibility Exercises

First, focus on the flexibility exercises. As stated before, there is a common pattern of muscular changes that is seen in lower back pain patients (lower crossed syndrome). It is most helpful to direct attention to the muscles indicated in this pattern, particularly the following:

a. Erector spinae
b. Hamstrings
c. Psoas
d. Tensor fasciae latae
e. Piriformis
f. Gastrocnemius/soleus

Demonstrate the correct procedure to the group and have them participate. Caution them not to be impatient or get frustrated and recommend establishing short-term, attainable goals such as a 1-inch improvement in flexibility in any given exercise in a 1-month time period. Flexibility does not just happen. It must be achieved.

Strengthening Exercises

Following stretching exercises the problem of muscle weakness should be addressed. The muscles most frequently identified with weakness in the low back pain patient are (a) abdominals, (b) gluteals, and (c) thigh.

Specific exercises for strengthening these muscles should be demonstrated and practiced. The position of strength should be reinforced at this point as strength in these muscles is necessary to effectively and safely accomplish this.

Exercises for Cardiovascular Fitness (Aerobic)

It has been shown that increased levels of fitness is one of the best ways of reducing the incidence of back injuries as well as a variety of other common musculoskeletal injuries. Thus, the improvement of cardiovascular performance is a necessary component in any injury prevention program. While it is not practical in the Back School setting to adequately address this area, certain general recommendations may be made:

a. Walking — a daily 20-minute brisk walk.
b. Bicycling — 20 minutes daily — the use of a stationary bicycle is particularly helpful and reduces the likelihood of inclement weather interfering with the exercise regimen.
c. Swimming — 20 minutes daily for those who have easy access to a swimming pool.
d. Attending soft (low-impact) aerobics classes — this should be considered as a target for those individuals who desire an organized exercise program.

Exercises for Balance and Coordination

One of the components that is often ignored in rehabilitation or prevention of musculoskeletal injuries is the development of balance and coordination. In recent years this has received a growing amount of attention. In all probability, time will not permit you to teach the necessary exercises to each individual in the class. It is suggested, however, that you evaluate the participants. You may find, in certain individuals, that a separate session is required specifically for this. The following is a suggested evaluation procedure that may easily be incorporated.

Evaluation

Have the group pair up and ask one member of the group to stand nearby the individual being tested in order to assist in case balance is poor. Ask the individual being tested to stand on one leg with arms at his/her side and eyes open, remain in this position for 15–20 seconds, and then close the eyes. You will often see a significant change in balance with the eyes closed as the individual is no longer able to rely on any visual assistance. This is often pronounced in individuals who have recurrent or chronic injuries of the foot and ankle. Repeat the procedure on the opposite leg. Change and test the second individual of the pair.

Rehabilitation of balance and coordination in patients with chronic injuries should be viewed as essential. The reader is referred to the "Exercises" section in Chapter 6.

SUMMARY

There are many different formats and styles of presentation of the information presented in the Back School. This chapter has attempted to provide some guidance in developing an organized approach for the individual considering establishing such a patient education program. The information provided in this chapter is based on information gathered from the literature, from my own personal conversations with others involved in the process of Back Schools, from personal visits to many operating Back Schools, and from my own experience with my patients. These thoughts represent my ideas and have been modified to fit my beliefs and personality. The reader is encouraged to add to, delete from, and modify these procedures in any way s/he sees fit. Good Luck.

References

1. Saunder HD. In: Isernhagen SJ, ed. *Work injury.* Rockville, MD: Aspen, 1988:27.
2. Mulry R. *Freedom from back pain.* Chicago: Nightingale-Conant, 1985.

6

Exercise Programs for Back Pain

One of the most commonly prescribed remedies for the patient with back pain is exercise. Patients have been encouraged to perform a variety of exercises in an effort to both hasten their recovery and to prevent future occurrences. The particular type of exercise regimen prescribed may vary from one practitioner to the next but the purpose is usually the same: i.e., to strengthen the weak muscles to aid in protecting the back.

It would be reasonable to assume that the doctor prescribing an exercise program would have a specific objective in mind. It is also reasonable to assume that the exercises prescribed would be tailored to the particular needs of the patient. Finally, it would be reasonable to provide assistance in training the patient to perform the exercises properly and to follow their progress over a period of time to determine the effectiveness, or ineffectiveness, of the prescribed regimen.

In actual fact, however, the "reasonable" steps indicated are seldom followed. Instead, too often the doctor prescribes the same exercise program for each of his/her patients with back pain (e.g., Williams flexion exercises). Rather than provide specific guidance and assistance in teaching the exercises to the patient, the doctor gives a patient a copy of the exercise regimen from a "prescription pad" and encourages the patient to "do these exercises at home." As far as follow-up is concerned, since the patient often feels better in a short period of time anyway, follow-up is deemed unnecessary or forgotten altogether. If the patient actually gets an individualized program with instructions and assistance, whether or not they actually do the exercises is influenced by a variety of factors (see

Chapter 8). It should hardly come as a surprise that many, including doctors and patients alike, consider exercise to be of little value.

The purpose of this chapter is to take a fresh look at the use of exercise in the total management of the back-injured individual. It must be appreciated that exercise is not to be considered curative. Rather, it is one part of the solution and is more helpful in some patients than in others. In addition, in order to be of any value, exercises must be performed. It is imperative that each patient understand the need for his/her exercise regimen and be properly schooled in the performance.

In Chapter 3 we listed multiple factors that individually or collectively contribute to the development of back pain. Obviously the contribution of any single factor will vary from patient to patient. An exercise program, if it is to be effective, must address each component and must focus on the individual factors deemed most important to the person performing the exercises. The following list provides the reader with a comparison of the contributing factors and the exercises suggested for each:

Contributing factors	Exercise program
1. Poor posture	Balance, coordination and postural exercises
2. Poor body mechanics	Mobility and strengthening exercises
3. Loss of flexibility	Mobility and flexibility exercises
4. Poor living and working habits	Flexibility and strengthening exercises
5. General decline in levels of fitness	Aerobics and conditioning exercises
6. Stress	Stress reduction and relaxation exercises

We will look at each category individually, but it should be clear that any given exercise may have more than one benefit. For instance, the knees to chest exercise increases the mobility of the hips and sacroiliac joints, stretches the erector spinae and gluteal muscles, and contributes to strengthening of the hip flexors and abdominal muscles. Specific exercise protocols will be identified (i.e., Williams flexion exercises and McKenzie's extension protocol).

It is sometimes a difficult task to decide which exercises are best for a particular patient. I recall a panel discussion that occurred at the Los Angeles College of Chiropractic in the spring of 1987. During the panel discussion several individuals were asked a variety of questions by the student audience. One of the questions was, "Which of the exercise programs was better for the low back patient, Williams or McKenzie's?" Each of us on the panel contributed our answer but the best response was provided by Dr. Scott Haldeman when he said: "I don't think it matters which the patient performs. What matters is that the patient do something for him/herself as early as possible."

SPECIFIC EXERCISE PROGRAMS

Prior to describing another series of suggested exercises it will be helpful to look at the more common exercise programs that have been used in the recent past. Of these, two stand out from the rest, the Williams flexion exercises and the McKenzie extension protocol. Both of these exercise programs, while somewhat contradictory in concept, have been successfully used for many years and have stood the test of time.

Williams Flexion Exercises

Anyone who has ever prescribed exercises for patients with low back pain is familiar with Williams flexion exercise program (1). The wide application of these exercises has, however, been largely without much scientific evidence to support their use. Williams felt that modern man developed back pain primarily due to an increase in the lordotic curve of the lumbar spine. His exercise program was developed, in large part, to reduce this lumbar lordosis and flatten the back. The rationale for the use of these exercises is:

1. To open the intervertebral foramen and facet joints to reduce compression on the nerve.
2. To stretch the hip flexors and back extensors that have overdeveloped due to the assumption of the upright posture.
3. To strengthen abdominal muscles and glutei.
4. To free the posterior fixation of the lumbosacral articulations.

The original program consisted of six simple exercises that are still in common use today (Fig. 6.1):

1. A partial sit-up performed with the knees bent (to strengthen the abdomen).
2. A pelvic tilt performed in the supine position (to strengthen the gluteal muscles and stretch the back extensors).

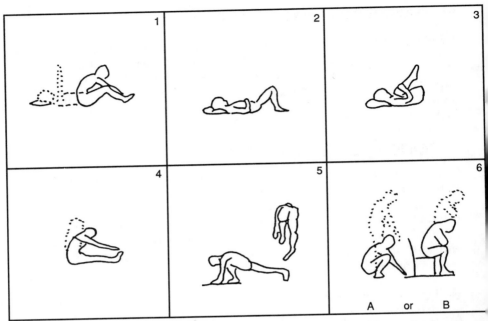

Figure 6.1. Williams flexion exercises. (Adapted from Williams PC. *Low back and neck pain: causes and conservative treatment.* Springfield: Charles C Thomas, 1974.)

3. The knees to chest performed in the supine position (to strengthen the abdominal muscles and to stretch the back extensors).
4. Low back and hamstring stretch performed in the seated, straight-leg position.
5. The fencers stretch or lunge (to stretch the hip flexors).
6. Squats performed either from full standing to a crouched position or to a seated position.

Over the years these exercises have become a part of nearly every exercise protocol for back pain. With the increased attention to lifting procedures and activities of daily living that has developed during the past two decades, the Williams exercises have continued. Currently the rationale is that strong abdominal muscles will protect the lumbar disc from extreme loads by producing an increase in the intra-abdominal pressure. While this line of reasoning is common, it is not altogether sound. The exercises, however, have proven to be a valuable part of a back exercise program.

McKenzie Extension Protocol

The second most widely utilized exercise protocol is more recently developed. Robin McKenzie (2), a New Zealand physical therapist views the development of back pain in a similar manner to Williams. McKenzie felt that posture, particularly sustained poor posture was a major contributing factor in its development. Unlike Williams, McKenzie felt that an increase in the lumbar lordosis was a beneficial element rather than a detriment and developed his exercise protocol in an effort to accentuate the forward curve in the lumbar spine.

The rationale for McKenzie's extension exercises includes the following:

1. The spine is better able to withstand compression stresses when the lordotic curve is maintained.
2. Extension unloads the disc and allows fluid intake.
3. There is a strong correlation between back muscle strength and lifting capacity.
4. Patients with back pain often demonstrate weakness of the back extensor muscles.
5. Prolonged flexion postures are often associated with the onset of back pain.

McKenzie's program consisted of a variety of exercises including:

1. the standing back bend,
2. the press-up,
3. sustained extension,
4. knees to chest,
5. standing toe touches,
6. standing hamstring stretch with leg on chair.

Comparison of Williams and McKenzie's Exercise Protocols

Williams' primary objective was to reduce the lumbar lordosis and he developed his exercise program to accomplish this task. McKenzie's goal, on the other hand, was to ultimately provide a full range of motion to the spine, including flexion and extension. The choice of which procedure to use, if any, is often based on the personal bias of the doctor rather than the evidence supporting the use of either. One study by Ponte et al. (3) compared the two treatment protocols to determine which was more effective in both decreasing pain and hastening a return of pain-free range of movement of the lumbar spine. The subjects included in the study fulfilled the following criteria: (a) between the ages of 21 and 55, (b) had observable limitation of active lumbar spine movement, (c) had low back pain of less then 3 weeks, and (d) had no history of serious low back pain within 6 months of this attack. In other words, one could anticipate that this group would typically respond in a short period of time. A total of 22 subjects were included in the study, 12 were assigned to the McKenzie protocol of treatment, and 10 received Williams flexion program. The results of this study indicated that the McKenzie protocol was significantly better than that of Williams in decreasing pain. 67% of the subjects receiving the McKenzie protocol were pain free at the end of treatment, whereas only 10% of the Williams group were completely free of pain at the post-treatment evaluation (3).

Jackson and Brown (4) provided an excellent review of current approaches to exercise. They state that exercise is often provided based on philosophical reasoning and tradition rather than on the basis of evidence that supports the particular exercises involved (4). Exercise programs are often seen as "flexion versus extension" or "strengthening versus mobility" instead of combinations of the various methods based on proper patient assessment. Back exercises may be utilized with the following goals:

1. To decrease pain.
2. To strengthen weak muscles.
3. To decrease mechanical stress to spinal structures.
4. To improve fitness levels to prevent injury.
5. To stabilize hypermobile segments.
6. To improve posture.
7. To improve mobility.
8. When all else fails.

EXERCISE PROGRAMS

In the following section we will describe a variety of exercise programs designed to address the specific problems that are encountered with the back pain patient. The exercises will be presented in order of appearance of the contributing factors rather than in order of their use. It is important to emphasize that each patient requires specific and individual evaluation and the variety and order of exercises prescribed for each should be based on the problems at hand, not on any formula.

Poor Posture

As stated earlier, the maintenance of a stressful posture, whether it be a flexed, forward-bent position, an extended, back-bent position, a twisted position, or some combination of the three, has a cumulative effect on the tissues of the spine. It would make sense that the patient who spends the day in a flexed, forward-bent position, who has a reduction of the lumbar lordosis or a flat-back, and who hurt his/her back in a flexed position will probably respond favorably to an initial round of exercises designed to restore the lumbar lordosis and minimize the flexed posture. On the other hand, the patient who has a sway back with an increased lordotic curve of the lumbar spine, who works with his/her back in an extended position, and who hurt his/her back while backward bending, will most likely respond to some flexion exercises.

A. Exercises to reduce the lumbar curve
   1. Knee(s) to chest
   2. Pelvic tilt
   3. Fencer's stretch
   4. Abdominal curls (partial sit-ups)
   5. Erector spinae stretch
   6. Hamstring stretch
   7. Gastrocnemius/soleus stretch
B. Exercises to increase the lumbar curve
   1. Standing back bend
   2. Press-up
   3. Leg lifts (prone)
   4. Flexion/extension on all fours
   5. Leg lifts (supine)
   6. Hamstring stretch
C. Exercises to improve balance and coordination

In addition to the exercises listed above, an important element in many patients with poor posture is the development of improper neuromuscular patterns. This may be, in part, due to a change in the proprioceptive input from injured joints and muscles. One of the areas that is currently receiving a great deal of attention in the rehabilitation of patients with musculoskeletal injuries, including back pain, is the assessment and treatment of muscle balance and coordination. The ability of the body to know the exact position of the joints and muscles is vital. Even if the muscles have adequate strength they cannot protect the joints and coordinate movement and balance if they do not get the proper messages. This may cause repetitive stress on muscles and joints and facilitate reinjury.

This is a simple test to evaluate the patient's balance and coordination:

1. Stand on one leg as relaxed as you can.
2. Steady yourself on one leg and close your eyes.
3. Repeat while standing on the other leg.

Use the following score sheet to grade the patient:

1. Excellent — can maintain steady balance for 30 seconds with eyes closed.
2. Very good — can maintain balance for 30 seconds with eyes closed but is unsteady.
3. Good — can maintain balance very steady with eyes open but unsteady with eyes closed.
4. Fair — can maintain balance for 30 seconds with eyes open but unsteady.
5. Poor — cannot maintain balance for 30 seconds.

The need for restoration of normal joint and muscle proprioception in an athlete is readily appreciated. The need for such improvement in a back-injured patient, while not as readily accepted, is every bit as necessary. Some of the more helpful tools to assist in this rehabilitation process are the rocker board, the wobble board (Fig. 6.2), the BAPS board, etc. The rocker board is perhaps the most easily utilized and readily available and a suggested protocol for its use follows:

Step 1. Open Kinetic Chain — begin with the patient in a seated position, eyes open, and progress through the following steps:
   a. 2 minutes rocking in an anterior to posterior direction.
   b. 2 minutes rocking in a side to side direction.
   c. Repeat with the opposite foot.
   d. Repeat the sequence with the eyes closed.
Step 2. Closed Kinetic Chain, Assisted — Follow the same procedure described in Step 1 with the patient in a supported

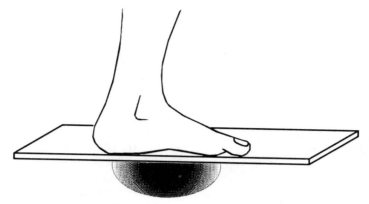

Figure 6.2. A wobble board.

weight-bearing position by having them place one hand against the wall to steady themselves.

Step 3. Closed Kinetic Chain, Unassisted — Follow the same procedure described above with the patient standing on both legs.

Step 4. Closed Kinetic Chain, Unassisted — Follow the procedure above with the patient standing on one leg at a time.

Helpful tips:

1. Use the rocker board on a carpeted surface so that it does not slip.
2. Focus attention on the task at hand.
3. Have the foot make as high an arch as possible when it contacts the rocker board.
4. Keep your body as relaxed as possible while doing this exercise.

A final component in restoring good posture is the use of a visualization technique that I learned several years ago from Dr. Leroy Perry, a Los Angeles chiropractor well-known for his work with athletes. According to Dr. Perry, this process was an important step in the rehabilitation of an injured athlete and often seemed to improve their athletic performance. This process is accomplished by asking the patient to envision four helium-filled balloons of their favorite color. One balloon is attached to the sternum, one to each shoulder, and one to the top of the head. The patient is instructed to allow the helium in the balloons to gently lift their frame into an upright posture. Whenever the patient sees something around them colored with their favorite color they are to envision the balloons lifting them up. While this exercise may seem rather silly, with practice it can make a substantial difference in the individuals carriage and is well worth the time and effort.

Poor Body Mechanics

The primary problem to be dealt with in this group is the improper functioning of the locomotor system (neuromusculoskeletal system). This dysfunction may be subdivided into three broad subcategories: (a) joints and muscles that are stiff and tight (flexibility), (b) joints and muscles that are weak and too loose (strengthening), and (c) joints and muscles that have lost their coordinated rhythmic functioning (balance and coordination).

Exercises to Increase Flexibility

Those joints and muscles that are stiff and tight will most likely respond to flexibility exercises that are designed to increase mobility. The following exercises are suggested for this category:

Joint flexibility exercises (Figs. 6.3–6.12):

1. Knee to chest
2. Knees to chest
3. Press up
4. Standing back bends
5. Trunk side-bending
6. Hip elevation
7. Toe touches
8. Squats
9. Trunk rotation
10. Flexion/extension (all fours)

Muscle stretches (Figs. 6.13–6.21):

1. Hamstring stretch
2. Erector spinae stretch
3. Quadriceps stretch
4. Piriformis stretch
5. Tensor fasciae latae (TFL) stretch
6. Gastrocnemius/soleus stretch
7. Psoas stretch
8. Hip adductors stretch
9. Upper back stretches

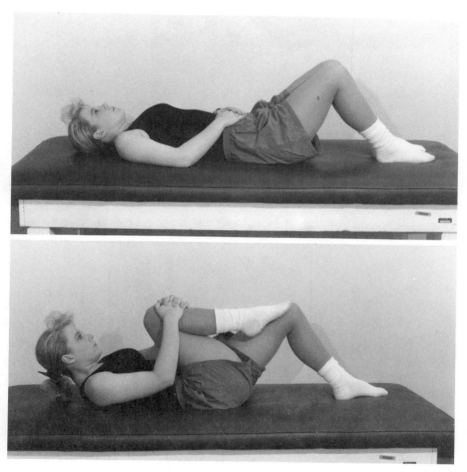

Figure 6.3. Knee to chest.

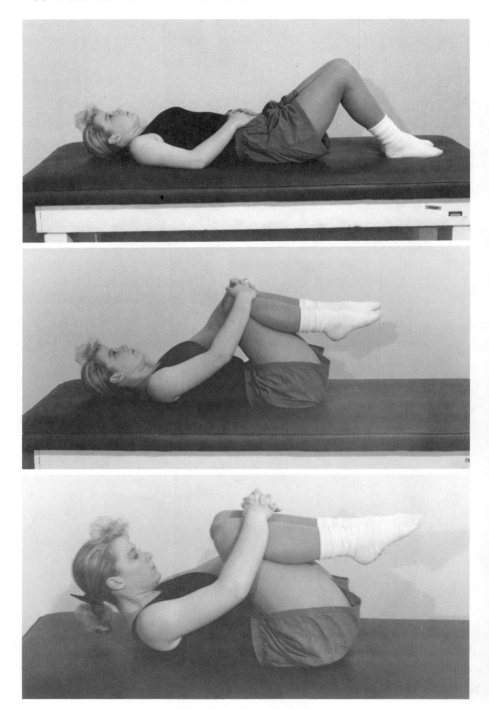

Figure 6.4. Knees to chest.

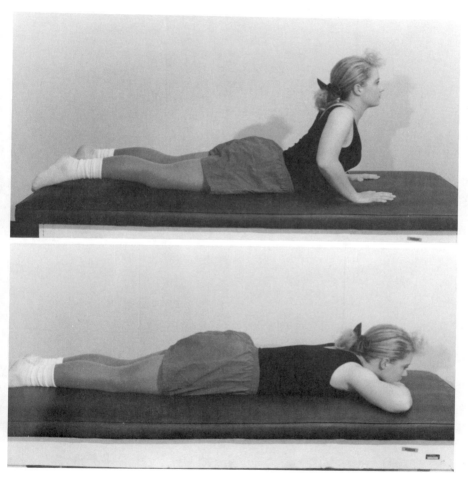

Figure 6.5. Press-up.

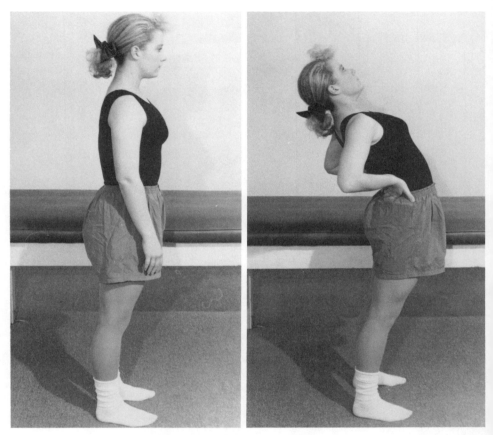

Figure 6.6. Standing back bends.

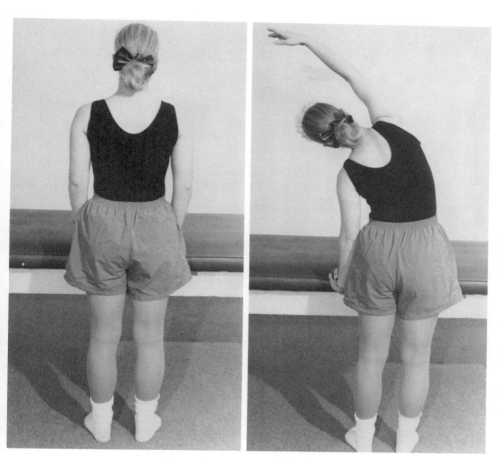

Figure 6.7. Trunk side-bending.

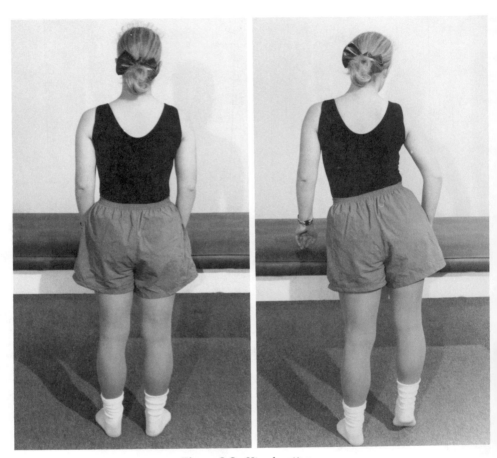

Figure 6.8. Hip elevation.

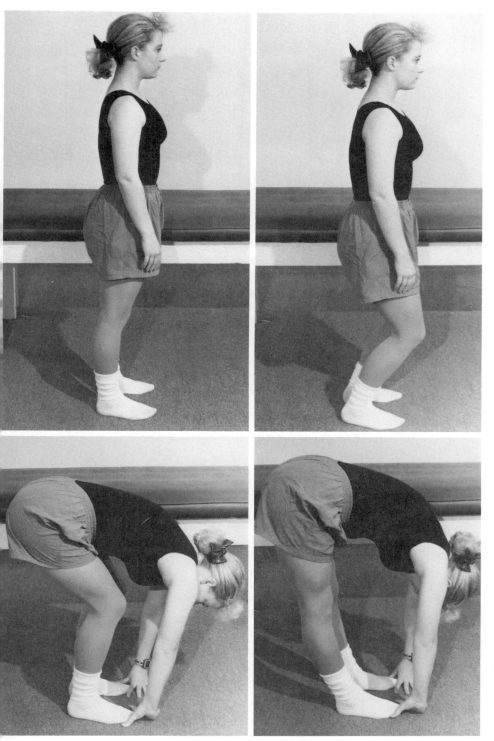

Figure 6.9. Toe touches.

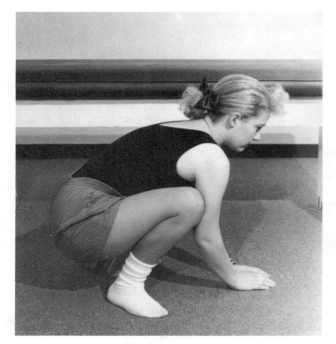

Figure 6.10. Squats.

   (i) Levator scapulae stretch
  (ii) Trapezius stretch
 (iii) Pectoralis stretch

I am of the opinion that the stretching exercises are, by far, the most important group of exercises for the back pain patient. The following are benefits of stretching (5):

a. Reduces muscle tension and makes the body feel more relaxed.
b. Helps coordination by allowing for freer and easier movement.
c. Increases range of motion.
d. Helps prevent injuries such as muscle strains.
e. Prepares for strenuous activities.
f. Helps develop body awareness.
g. Promotes circulation.

It is important to emphasize to the patient that any stretching and/or mobility exercises should be performed slowly. The patient

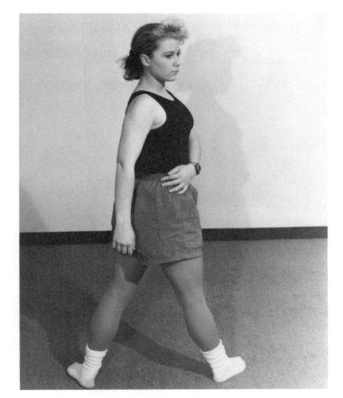

Figure 6.11. Trunk rotation.

should not bounce and should expect a slow but gradual change over a period of time. Flexibility is only earned with perseverance.

Stretching Procedure

When beginning a stretching regimen spend 10–30 seconds in a gentle, easy stretch. Go to the point of mild tension and relax as you hold the stretch. If the exercise is performed properly the feeling of tension should gradually disappear as the position is held. If not, gradually reduce the tension to a more comfortable position.

Follow this first easy, relaxed stretch with a more moderate stretch by moving just a little further into the stretched position. Hold this new position for another 10–30 seconds and ease off if it becomes uncomfortable. Be sure to breathe slowly and fully as the

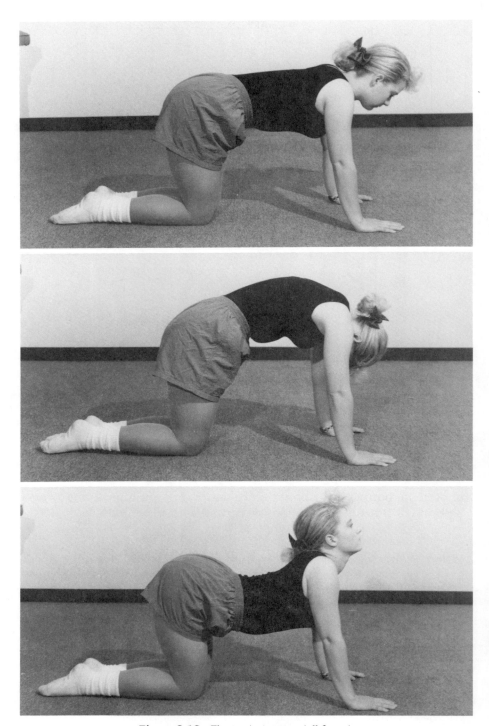

Figure 6.12. Flexion/extension (all fours).

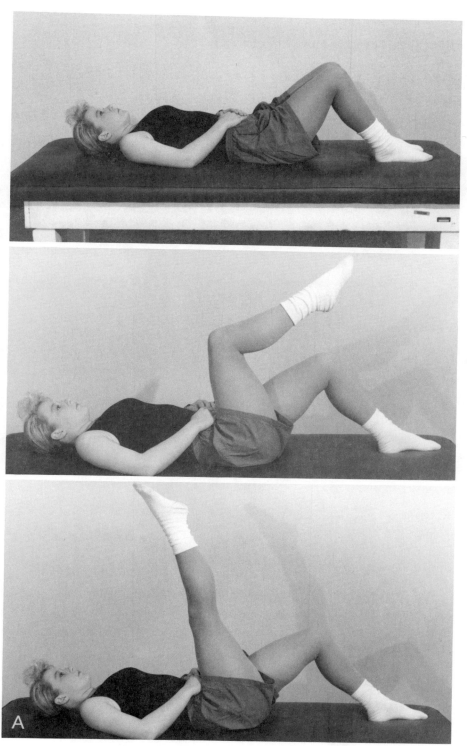

Figure 6.13. Hamstring stretch — supine (**A**) and standing (**B**).

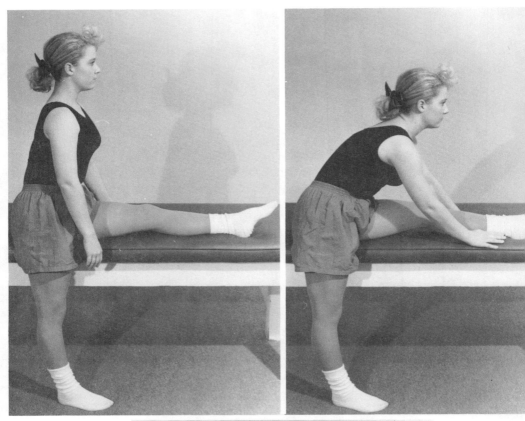

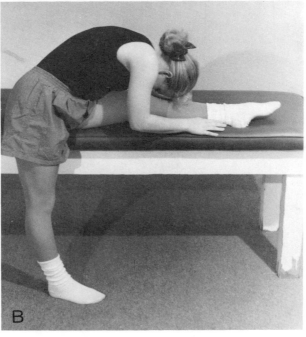

B

Figure 6.13. *Continued.*

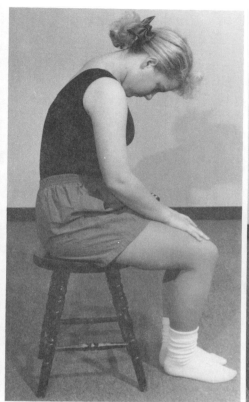
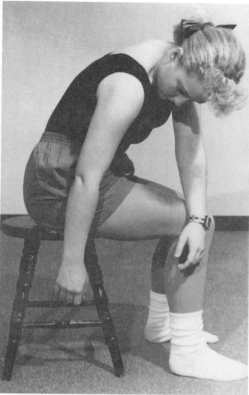
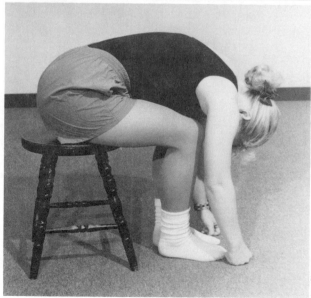

Figure 6.14. Erector spinae stretch.

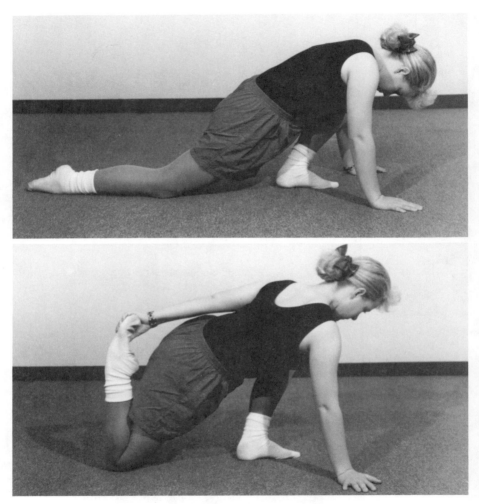

Figure 6.15. Quadriceps stretch.

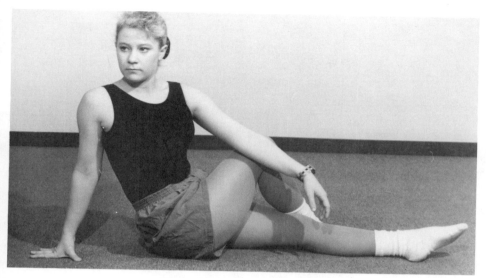

Figure 6.16. Piriformis stretch.

stretch is performed. Once completed, move around to loosen up further.

Post-isometric Relaxation Technique

One method that can facilitate the stretching exercises is the use of the post-isometric relaxation techniques. This is termed a "muscle energy technique" and has been utilized for many years as a method of attaining greater stretch of stiff muscles. The post-isometric relaxation method involves the following steps:

1. Position the muscle that is to be stretched near its physiological limit. The muscle should be tight but not stressed.
2. Hold the muscle in the position and ask the patient to apply a gentle contraction of the muscle for 5–10 seconds. Your resistance to the contraction provides an isometric contraction to the muscle. It should not be allowed to shorten during this phase. It is important to point out that a gentle contraction, perhaps only 10 or 20% of the total muscle strength, is all that is necessary.
3. After the period of isometric contraction ask the patient to relax. It is helpful at this point to take a deep breath and exhale. During the exhalation (relaxation phase), gently stretch the muscle. You may repeat the procedure 3 or 4 times at a setting.

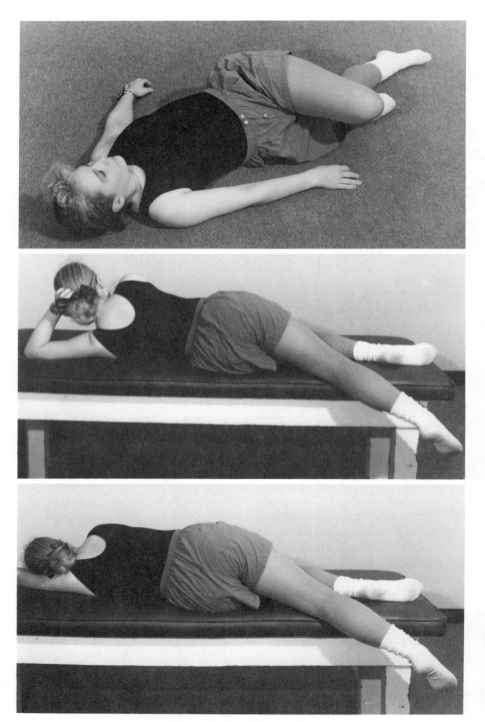

Figure 6.17. TFL stretch.

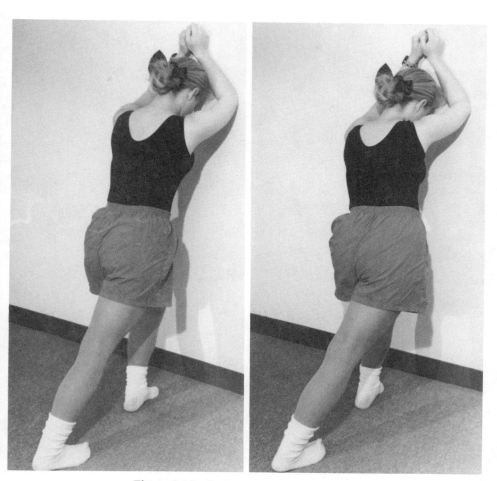

Figure 6.18. Gastrocnemius/soleus stretch.

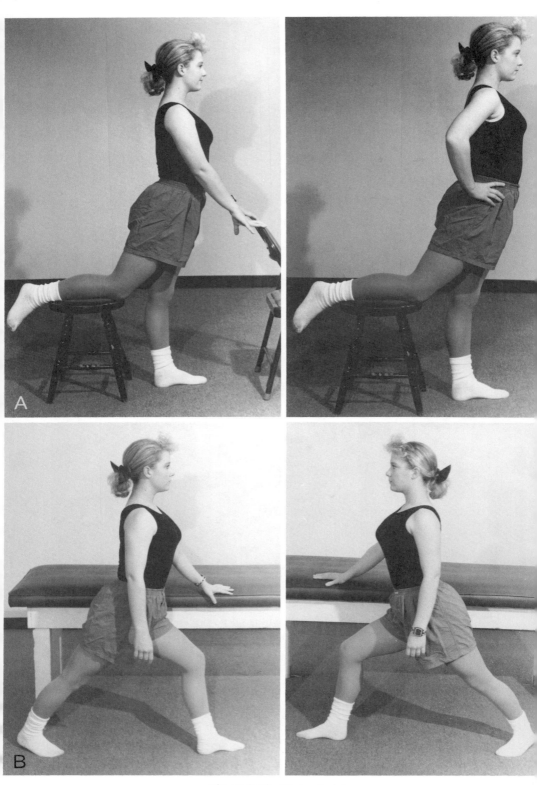

Figure 6.19. Psoas stretch.

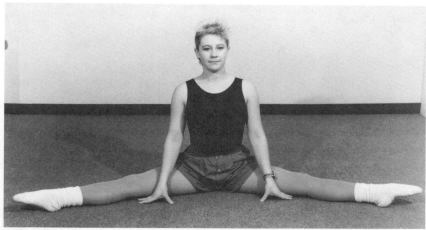

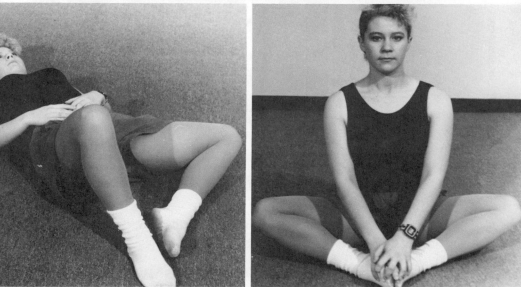

Figure 6.20. Hip adductors stretch.

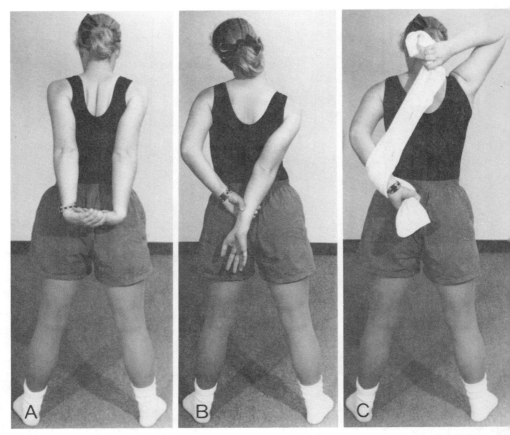

Figure 6.21. Upper back stretches: levator scapulae stretch (**A**), trapezius stretch (**B**), pectoralis stretch (**C**).

Strengthening Exercises

Most often when exercise programs are recommended they fall into either strengthening or conditioning exercises. These should be performed only after the flexibility and mobility exercises have been accomplished and may be followed by more stretching. The following list provides a common variety of exercises that are specifically designed to increase muscle strength (Figs. 6.22–6.31):

1. Abdominal curls — rectus abdominis
2. Pelvic tilt — gluteal muscles
3. Back bends (prone) — erector spinae

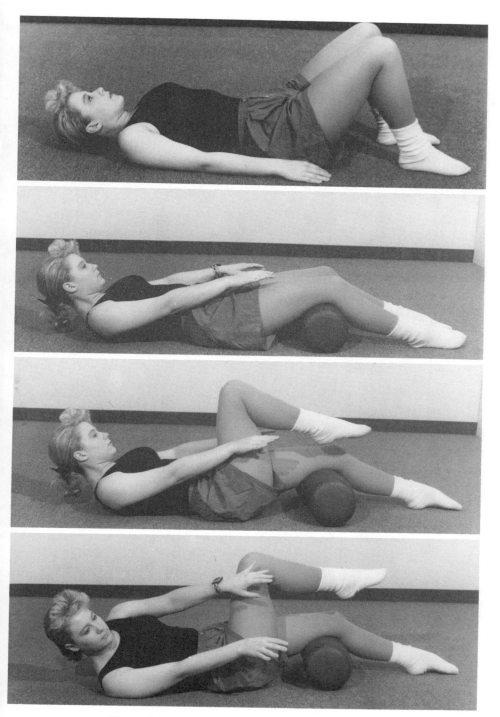

Figure 6.22. Adbominal curls — rectus abdominis.

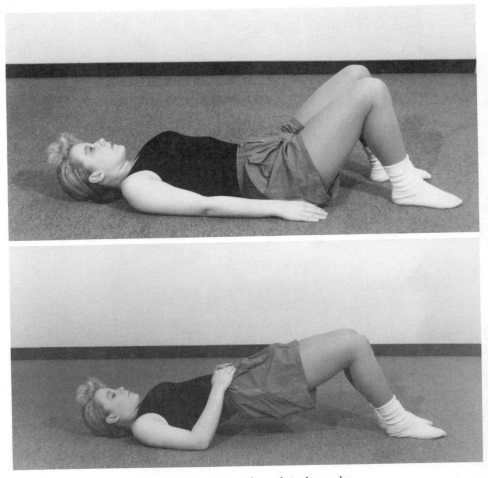

Figure 6.23. Pelvic tilt — gluteal muscles.

4. Leg raises (supine) — quadriceps and psoas
5. Leg raises (prone) — hip extensors
6. Toe raises — gastroc/soleus
7. Hip abduction — TFL and piriformis
8. Rhomboid exercises — scapular stabilizers
9. Wall squats — quadriceps
10. Buttocks squeezing — gluteal muscles

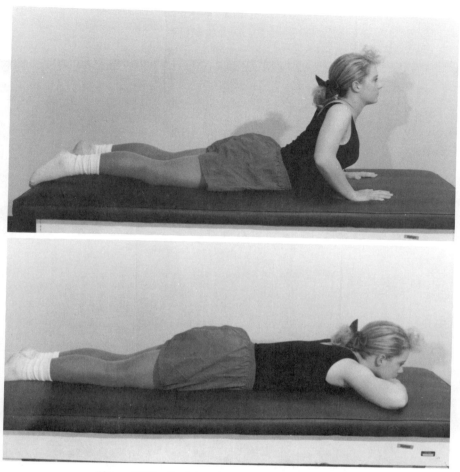

Figure 6.24. Back bends (prone) — erector spinae.

The general sequence for strengthening weak muscles should be as follows:

Step 1. *Isometric Exercise Program.* Many of these, such as the pelvic tilt, may be safely performed during the acute episode of back pain. It is probably helpful for many reasons, not the least of which is the psychological aspect, to begin some type of exercise program as early as possible.

Step 2. *Isotonic Exercise Program.* After a conditioning period of a few days to several weeks the patient should begin isotonic

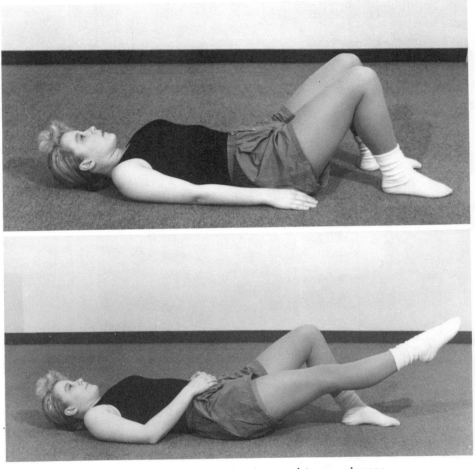

Figure 6.25. Leg raises (supine) — quadriceps and psoas.

exercises using only the weight of the body. The addition of free weights may be used as the patient progresses and improves if desired. This program, while not as technologically advanced as those using mechanically assisted devices, will be more than adequate for most patients.

Step 3. *Isokinetic Exercise Program.* If the doctor and the patient agree, if the nature of the injury warrants, and if access to equipment is not a problem, the patient may next move to isokinetic equipment such as the Cybex machines. While

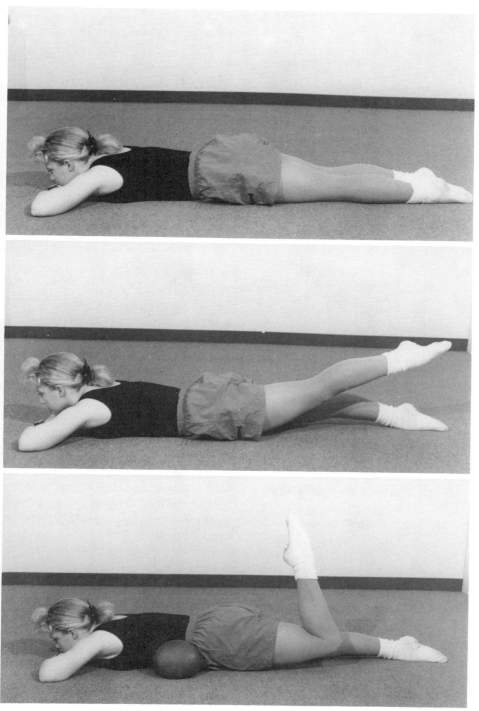

Figure 6.26. Leg raises (prone) — hip extensors.

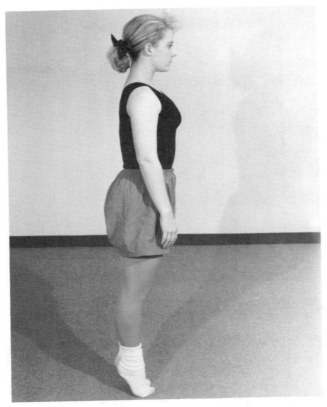

Figure 6.27. Toe raises — gastrocnemius/soleus.

these procedures are costly from both a financial and time factor they offer several distinct advantages: 1) equipment may also be used to evaluate the patient's strength, 2) the information gathered may provide an objective baseline for charting patient progress, and 3) patient feedback is good (some patients appreciate the use of such modern and sophisticated equipment).

Balance and Coordination

Many mechanical problems in the musculoskeletal system are associated with changes in the balance and coordination of the body parts. As stated earlier, it is easy to appreciate the need for good balance and coordination in the injured athlete (dancer, gymnast, downhill skier, etc.). The demands on the injured worker (industrial

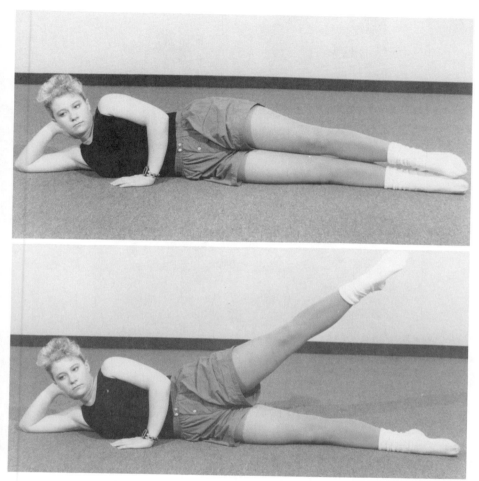

Figure 6.28. Hip abduction — TFL and piriformis.

athlete) are just as great. The exercises used for rehabilitation in this area utilize the wobble board and the reader is referred to the section of this chapter on "Poor Posture."

Loss of Flexibility

The maintenance of flexibility, in my opinion, is synonymous with the maintenance of health. It is no coincidence that the sedentary lifestyle is associated with so many degenerative conditions, includ-

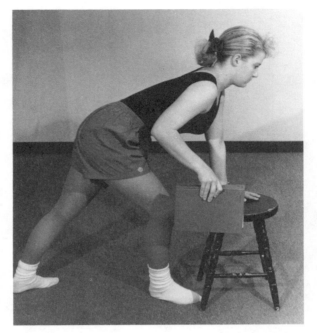

Figure 6.29. Rhomboid exercises — scapular stabilizers.

ing back pain. The restoration of flexibility of the musculoskeletal system is, perhaps, the most important aspect of the rehabilitation of the back pain patient and should become a major priority of treatment. While the doctor may assist the patient in beginning a flexibility program, ultimately the patient must accept responsibility for this important component. The specific exercises used for restoring flexibility to the back pain patient are described earlier under the heading "Poor Body Mechanics."

Poor Living and Working Habits

The appropriate use of the body during normal daily activities is dependent upon several factors: 1) knowledge of proper lifting methods and other ADL, etc., 2) adequate strength and coordination of muscles, and 3) adequate joint and muscle flexibility. The exercises used for these purposes are addressed in the sections on "Poor Body Mechanics" and "Poor Posture." The knowledge of proper lifting techniques, etc., is addressed in Chapter 5.

A recent development in the rehabilitation of the disabled or

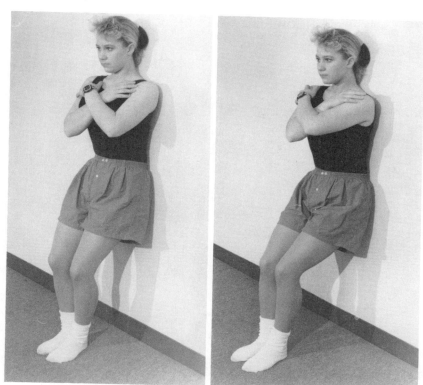

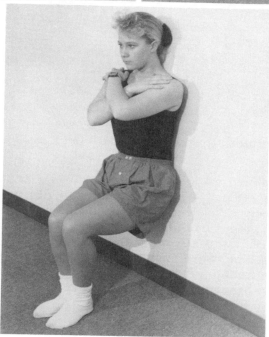

Figure 6.30. Wall squats — quadriceps.

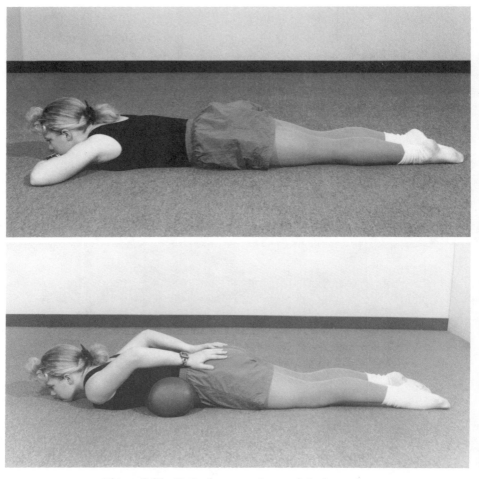

Figure 6.31. Buttocks squeezing — gluteal muscles.

chronically injured worker is the use of "Work Hardening." This consists of specifically designed work stations that provide an "on-the-job" setting for teaching the individual appropriate use of his/her body, proper tool utilization, and safe working habits. In some instances, it is used to teach an injured worker a different task or occupation. The use of such "work hardening" involves a great deal of time and effort and it is not the focus of this text. The reader is referred to other sources listed at the end of this chapter for more information on this topic.

General Decline in Levels of Fitness

It is this area that is often overlooked in the back injured patient. The individual who has a relatively sedentary lifestyle often assumes a more sedentary life during the post-injury phase. The individual in pain may frequently avoid activities that s/he may otherwise engage in due to the pain. Consider the office worker whose only exercise comes from an occasional game of golf and doing yard work around the house. While mowing the lawn on the weekend, s/he injures his/her back. S/he is told by the doctor to reduce activities to a minimum for the next few weeks and to rest in bed whenever possible. Any attempts to continue normal activities are met with a return of the back pain and the injured individual quickly learns to hire a teenage neighbor to mow the lawn. The occasional game of golf is replaced with Saturday afternoons spent watching college football on television. The longer the individual remains inactive, the more difficult it will be to return to any semblance of physical activity.

Interest in promoting general health and fitness for the back pain patient is growing. Such interest began, largely as a result of the classic study of firefighters by Cady et al. (6). A general conclusion that was drawn from this study, a conclusion that has been borne out by others is that, rather than the work being a cause of back injury, the fitness of the worker for the work may be a greater factor.

Exercises designed for improving cardiovascular fitness and endurance as well as musculoskeletal fitness play a major role in the complete rehabilitation of the back pain patient. Such exercises should involve some type of aerobic activity and appropriate cardiovascular screening is recommended prior to initiating such a program. The conditioning exercise program: 1) should range from 30 to 40 minutes and should include both a warm-up and a cool-down period, 2) should be performed 3–5 times weekly, 3) should be regular in performance (in certain areas modifications must be made to account for inclement weather), and 4) should be acceptable to the patient (identify an activity the patient enjoys). The following types of aerobic activities are suggested:

1. Walking and jogging. Walking is perhaps the best overall exercise and is safe for most people. Care must be taken to select an appropriate pair of walking shoes, preferably with some type of cushioning effect and to select an appropriate, and safe walking surface. Jogging, on the other hand should probably be discouraged for most back pain patients.

2. Swimming. Swimming provides an excellent non-weight bearing aerobic activity. Some patients may be uncomfortable while swimming due to the extension of the lumbar spine. This may be easily remedied by using a flotation device around the waist.

3. Bicycling. Bicycling is associated with prolonged sitting and a sustained flexed, forward-bent posture. Consequently, not every patient will benefit as much from a cycling program. However, the use of a stationary cycle can be an effective addition to the walker or swimmer during inclement weather and may break up the routine and add enjoyment.

4. Jumping rope. This exercise, while providing a significant amount of cardiovascular activity is associated with repetitive loading of the spine and is not recommended for most back pain patients.

5. Dance aerobics. Care must be taken to select a program that is tailored to the patients needs. Many such programs involve a great deal of bending and twisting and may create more problems than they resolve.

SUMMARY

In conclusion, the appropriate use of an exercise program that is tailored to the individual needs of the patient and that is designed with the patient's lifestyle in mind is one of the most useful components in any back care rehabilitation or prevention program. The use of preprinted exercise forms that are given to the patient along with advice to "do these at home" are, in all probability, a waste of time. If this text accomplished nothing else other than direct you to re-evaluate the exercises that you ask your back pain patients to perform, it has been a worthwhile project.

References

1. Williams PC. *Low back and neck pain: causes and conservative treatment.* Springfield: Charles C Thomas, 1974:35–43.
2. McKenzie RA. *The lumbar spine: mechanical diagnosis and therapy.* New Zealand: Spinal Publications, 1981.
3. Ponte JD, Gail JJ, Kent BE. A preliminary report on the use of the McKenzie protocol versus Williams protocol in the treatment of low back pain. *J Ortho Sports Phys Ther* Sept./Oct. 1984:130–139.
4. Jackson CP, Brown MD. Is there a role for exercise in the treatment of patients with low back pain? *Clin Orthop Relat Res* 1983;179:39–45.
5. Anderson R. *Stretching.* Bolinas, CA: Shelter Publications, 1980.
6. Cady LD, Bischoff DP, O'Connell ER, et al. Strength and fitness and subsequent back injuries in firefighters. *J Occup Med* 1979;21:269.

7

Preventing Back Pain in Industry

The chiropractic profession has only recently begun to involve itself in the industrial arena. Unfortunately, the motivation for this is often to increase the share of the worker's compensation "pie" and to promote the benefits of chiropractic treatment rather than to provide a solid prevention program for industry. With the continuing rapid escalation in the costs of back pain and in the overall costs of health care, industry must utilize new and creative ways of reducing expenditures in these areas.

In this chapter we will discuss the various components involved in preventing back problems in the work place. These include:

a. Identifying the occupational risk factors associated with low back pain.
b. Identifying the individual risk factors associated with low back pain.
c. Evaluating the prospective employee (preemployment screening).
d. Job design and ergonomics.
e. Education and training programs for employees and employers.

OCCUPATIONAL RISK FACTORS

Material Handling

Occupations, particularly those involving repetitive lifting of heavy objects, have long been associated with the development of low back pain. As early as 2780 BC an ancient Egyptian reported back pain in workers during the construction of a pyramid (1). Since that time extensive studies have been performed in Sweden, Great Britain, Canada, and the United States in an attempt to identify hazardous occupations (2–5). It is generally agreed that manual material handlers represent the single largest group in the work force who are affected by back pain (6). Some claim that as much as 50% of all work-related back injuries are the result of such material handling. Of these injuries, lifting has been associated with 37–49%, pushing objects with 9–16%, pulling with 6–9%, and carrying with 5–8% (7). Many occupations such as forestry workers, miners, railroad workers, truck drivers, and nurses have been linked to higher incidence of occurrence. Hult (8) showed not only a higher incidence of injury in heavy industry workers when compared to those in light industry, but a statistically higher incidence of severe back pain (8). Faced with all of the data it is reasonable to assume that a major risk factor is the occupation itself. Those individuals who are consistently required to lift objects are at higher risk for back pain than those who are not (Fig. 7.1).

Vibration

In addition to material handling, many other factors appear to play a significant role in the development of on-the-job back problems. Of these perhaps the presence of some type of vibrational stress is most important. The most commonly reported effects of industrial vibration are low back pain and degenerative changes in the lumbar spine (8). Some claim that the long term exposure to vibration may be every bit as harmful to the lumbar spine as handling heavy objects. It might be argued that workers in occupations that involve both the handling of heavy objects and constant vibrational stresses (such as truck drivers who also load and unload their trucks) are predestined for low back pain.

It has long been recognized that truck drivers have a high incidence of back pain. Kelsey (9) notes that truck drivers are 4 times more likely to have a disc herniation than the general population (10). Several other occupations fall into the high risk category for vibration: aircraft pilots (particularly helicopter pilots), agriculture workers (especially those driving tractors), construction workers (earth-moving equipment), and transportation workers (taxi, train, bus, and truck drivers) (9).

Posture

A third risk category is the posture assumed while on the job. Jobs requiring prolonged stooping appear to be at greater risk. Afacan (10) noted that the incidence of work absenteeism in coal miners

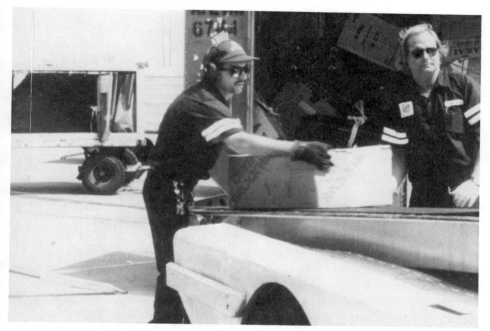

Figure 7.1. Back injuries are a common occurrence in the workplace.

was significantly higher in those who worked underground than in those who worked on the surface, presumably due to the constant stooping demanded by the low ceilings in the coal mine (10). A similar observation was made by Undeutsch et al. (11) in aircraft baggage handlers who are frequently in awkward positions in the hold of an aircraft. Taller workers (those over 178 cm) had a higher incidence (73%) when compared with shorter workers (those under 164 cm) who had only a 53% occurrence (11). This again is presumably due to the increased stooping (Fig. 7.2).

My own observations in working with aircraft ground crews support the observations of Undeutsch. After spending several minutes standing in the baggage hold of a DC-10 airliner with a ceiling height of approximately 5 feet 8 inches, my 5 feet 10 inch frame became more and more uncomfortable. Of all the workers I observed, those under 5 feet 6 inches who were able to stand erect in the hold appeared to be the most comfortable.

Many on-the-job factors may, individually or collectively, add to the risk of back problems developing. One study of nurses concluded

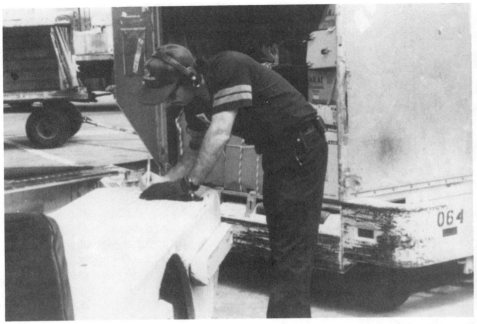

Figure 7.2. The stooped, forward-bent posture that is common to many workplaces is a contributing factor in the development of back pain.

that four factors were positively associated with injury: job category, lifting, work activity, and previous history of back complaints (12).

INDIVIDUAL RISK FACTORS

Many individual factors add to the likelihood of future back pain. Such factors as age, sex, height, weight, and physical fitness have been studied.

Age

It is generally agreed that age, while important, is not inherently an etiologic factor. It is apparent, however, that there is a relationship between age and back pain. The typical back pain patient is somewhere between the ages of 25 and 65 with a peak in the 55–64-year range. The prevalence for sciatica is slightly less, 45–54 years. Most back trouble begins in the third decade with few cases beginning before the age of 20 and the number of new cases declining after 30 (13). Kirkaldy-Willis (14) shows a peak incidence of approximately 55 years of age with a declining rate thereafter. With this high incidence occurring during the middle years, those associated with the most productive employment, it is no wonder that the worker disabled with a back injury, becomes such a costly statistic.

In my opinion, the relative lack of reported back injuries prior to the age of 20 is misleading. Most chiropractors and physicians who see children in a general practice realize that they, too, have back problems. Lewit (15) describes a study of children between the ages of 3 and 6, some 30% of whom already had a history of back pain. Mierau et al. (16) reported a similar study of teenagers in which the incidence of back pain was about the same. In all probability, many of the back problems that develop in the young individual respond with little or no care and are dismissed as unimportant. As we shall see later, one of the most significant predictors of back pain is a past history of back problems and these early, seemingly benign conditions should not be overlooked.

The relationship between age and degenerative changes in the spine is clear. As we age, the disc tends to lose height, osteophytes form, and there may be accompanying narrowing of the intervertebral foramen and even the spinal foramen. What the relationship is between these degenerative changes and the presence of back pain is not as clear. It may seem puzzling that while the degenerative cycle continues with advancing years the incidence of back pain peaks, only to decline with advancing age. Perhaps this decline in back symptoms is due to a general reduction in physical activity and work-related stress that often accompanies the more senior laborer.

Height and Weight

Kirkaldy-Willis (14) states that body type does not seem to correlate with the occurrence of back pain. Mandell et al. (6) claim the book is still open in this area. They cite studies such as those of Undeutsch (11), Gyntelberg (17), and Hrubec (18), that show a significant positive correlation between height and occurrence of back pain. Other studies such as those of Manning (19) and Brennan (20) show no clear correlation. Heliovarra (21) implicated height as a positive predictive factor. In his study, the risk of herniation in the tallest men and women was 2 and 4 times greater, respectively, than their shorter counterparts (those 10 cm shorter) (21).

At first glance these studies may appear to be conflicting. It might be concluded, however, that height only becomes a factor at a certain point and might be more of a factor when associated with jobs requiring increased stooping. This would be consistent with observations of workers in underground mine shafts and airline baggage holds.

Weight, it seems, does not have a strong predictive value except, perhaps, as it relates to reduced levels of fitness.

Sex

No strong correlation appears in regard to the sex of the patient. There does, however, appear to be a difference in the treatment between men and women. Sprangfort (22) showed men 2 times as likely to undergo surgery for disc herniations than women, while Kelsey and Ostfeld (23) stated that for the same degree of symptoms men are more likely to undergo surgery than women.

Previous History

A most important indicator of future back pain is a history of previous episodes. Many studies have shown a high recurrence rate and Chaffin and Park (24) cite previous incidence as a significant risk factor. As stated earlier, while back pain is considered self-limiting and is associated with a rapid recovery in most individuals, it is also associated with a high recurrence rate, perhaps as high as 95% (25).

Physical Fitness

Of utmost importance to the prevention of injury is the general fitness of the worker. Perhaps more important than the job itself is the fitness of the worker for the job. As demonstrated by Cady et al. (26) in his 1979 study of firefighters there is a direct relationship between levels of fitness, emphasizing cardiovascular stamina, and the incidence of back pain. Simply put, the healthier the worker the less likely s/he is to be injured. This fact should not be viewed lightly by anyone interested in reducing the occurrence of health problems, including back pain, in industry. The promotion of health and wellness rather than the treatment of disease has always been a major premise of the chiropractic profession, and such efforts pay large dividends to the employer, the employees, and to the industrial consultant.

Strength

Muscle strength has also positively correlated to back pain. Alston (27) claimed that those patients with chronic back pain also had a general weakness of truck musculature. A study by Biering-Sorenson (28) found a lower isometric endurance of back muscles, tight extensors of the back, and tight hamstrings in men with back pain. Suzuki et al. (29) demonstrated that trunk flexors were typically weaker in back pain patients than in controls but found no such relationship for trunk extensors (29). On the other hand, Nachemson (30) and others could find no evidence linking back pain with trunk muscle weakness. Timm (31) indicates that the process of gathering trunk strength data is complex and varied and this factor may contribute to the varied results.

As will be discussed later in this chapter, it may not be useful to use trunk muscle strength alone as a predictor. As part of a general evaluation of a worker's health and his/her fitness for a particular job, however, it may be one of many useful tools.

Smoking

Along with all of the other health problems associated with cigarette smoking, it is clear that smokers have a significantly higher rate of back pain and intervertebral disc prolapse. Some suggest this may be due to the chronic cough so often associated with smoking (32, 33). Others feel it may be due to the accompanying reduction in bone mineral content similar to that seen with osteoporosis (34). Or perhaps it may be associated with a reduction in blood flow to the vertebral body and disruption of the tenous nutrient supply to the intervertebral disc (35). Whatever the mechanism, studies demonstrate that smokers have a considerably greater chance of developing back pain than nonsmokers.

Psychosocial Risk Factors

Much evidence supports the contention that the degree of tissue damage, disc herniation, degenerative changes seen on x-ray, etc. do not directly correlate with the degree of pain and discomfort. Rather, the perception of pain and the reaction to pain by the patient may be influenced by a variety of factors including the degree of emotional stress, job satisfaction, level of education, and the presence of secondary gain. A study by Vallfors (36) listed the following factors as statistically significant:

Unmarried or divorced
Unsatisfactory housing
Spouse working outside the home

Dissatisfied with work mates
Greater frequency of neurosis, migraine, ulcers
Alcohol and tobacco use

It would appear that back pain is more of a detriment to low-income workers in unfulfilling occupations who are somehow dissatisfied with their lives and jobs. Dr. Reed Phillips, Director of Research at Los Angeles College of Chiropractic, has referred to back pain as a "social disease" and, in many respects, I agree.

It has been stated by some that educational level may be the most significant risk factor of any. Deyo and Tsui-Wu (37) evaluated 1516 back pain patients and found that they were generally older, less educated, and with less income than a control group who had no history of back pain. Deyo claimed that educational level is also a general indicator of degree of job satisfaction, job strenuousness, and degree of job input (37).

EVALUATING THE PROSPECTIVE EMPLOYEE

From an ideal point of view one of the most useful aspects involved in preventing back injuries in the industrial setting is the process involved in identifying the individual who is at risk prior to placing him/her in an occupation that s/he is physically unsuited for. In other words, injuries may be prevented by selecting the best worker for a given task and selecting the best task for a given worker.

In an industry such as professional athletics this preselection is of utmost importance. Before an athlete is considered for a professional football team, for example, he must meet certain physical requirements such as weight, speed, strength, and stamina. The physical requirements for a center or tackle are quite different from that demanded of a placekicker or a tight end. Prior to issuing a prospective employee a contract the team medical staff gives the athlete a thorough physical examination. Periodically we hear of a young athlete who is rejected due to some anomaly such as a congenitally stenotic cervical spine, a spina bifida, or ligamentous laxity in the knee. This physical exam is accepted as a necessary preemployment step in athletes.

Similar physical evaluations are performed in selected other industries such as airline pilots and astronauts. Why similar considerations are not routinely given when hiring an "industrial athlete" who is going to work in a heavy industry that carries a high injury rate is complex. Sometimes the reason may simply be a lack of awareness on the part of the employer. In other instances the "up-front" costs of such a physical exam may appear too large to a company already financially strapped. This may be particularly true for a company with a high turnover rate of new employees.

A more complicated reason may be the legal ramifications involved. Take, for example, an occupation requiring a combination of strength and stamina that perhaps involves the lifting of heavy objects high overhead. It would seem that a strong, tall person would be at somewhat of an advantage over a small, short individual. Suppose, however, that a 90-pound female who stands 4 feet 10 inches applies for the job. Suppose also that this divorced mother of four is the sole support for her children and that this may be the best paying job in town that she could hope to get. What are the legal and moral issues involved? Obviously she should not be denied every opportunity to support her family. To deny her such a chance based on her physical size is unfair. On the other side, however, it is equally unfair to both the individual and to the employer (who must pay for her health care) to place her in an occupation in which she is physically at risk.

To complicate this problem even more, as stated earlier in this chapter, there does not appear to be much agreement on which factors indeed are positive predictors of future back pain.

History

One of the most significant indicators of future back pain is a past history of back problems. Lloyd and Troup (38) stated that a history which includes the following increases the likelihood of recurrence with each additional factor:

a. A history of two or more episodes.
b. A past injury resulting from a fall.
c. A history of residual leg pain.
d. Lost work time in excess of five weeks.

With this in mind, an important part of the screening process should include a comprehensive and accurate medical history with particular emphasis on the back. Any problems identified should be thoroughly recorded and investigated. As part of this history some type of psychosocial evaluation would be helpful. This will be discussed in greater detail later in this chapter.

Pre-employment Physical Examination

General Health

With Cady's (26) study of firefighters in mind an important component of any pre-employment physical screening should incorporate an evaluation of overall health, including cardiovascular fitness.

Strength Testing

In addition to a general physical examination, the use of various strength testing procedures has recently become popular. Chaffin and Andersson (39) provide the following general guidelines for strength testing:

1. The measurements should accurately estimate a specific, definable, human motor function; that is, they should provide well-correlated and unbiased estimates of the function of interest.
2. The data should be repeatable under prescribed conditions.
3. The measurements should provide estimates of the limits of function; that is, distinguish between normal and abnormal.
4. The measurement system should not alter the function being estimated.
5. The measurement system should be safe to use.
6. The measurement system should be practical; that is, easy to set up and use, insensitive to outside influences, and inexpensive.

Isometric Muscle Strength Testing

Muscle strength testing incorporates primarily the use of isometric (static) and isokinetic (dynamic) procedures. Mandell et al. (6) claim that, based on some of the work of Chaffin at the University of Michigan, isometric testing can predict the likelihood of future back problems. They cite several studies that classified workers in the following groups:

a. Understressed — employees with a high strength capability.
b. Considerably stressed — employees in jobs that closely taxed their strength capabilities.
c. Overstressed — employees who were unable to demonstrate as much strength as their job required.

The results over an extended period of time indicated that as the requirement of strength in the performance of a particular task approached or exceeded the actual isometric strength of the worker the back injury rates and severity rates increased by 300% (40). Studies by other investigators have yielded similar results (41, 42). The advantages of isometric strength testing are;

a. The test seems to have a reasonable predictive value.
b. The testing is relatively easy to perform.
c. It is easy to duplicate specific tasks in a testing setting.
d. The tests are relatively inexpensive to perform.
e. There is good reliability and reproducibility between testors.
f. The tests are safe to perform.

The primary disadvantages of isometric strength testing are:

a. They only test one plane of movement at a time.
b. The tests do not incorporate joint movement.
c. The tests do not allow for changes in posture, joint loading, and muscle length/tension ratios.
d. The tests do not account for acceleration and deceleration of body segments (6).

Isokinetic Muscle Strength Testing

A second type of muscle testing procedure incorporates the use of isokinetic devices such as the Cybex "Liftask" (Fig. 7.3), "TEF" (trunk extension/flexion), and "TOR" (trunk rotation) units. These procedures provide a more realistic assessment of the actual lifting risk by incorporating measurement throughout a range of motion. They also provide a reliable and repeatable assessment that has good predictive value. The primary disadvantage of such isokinetic testing is the relatively high cost. Compared to the cost of a single severe back injury, however, the cost may be easily justified.

With regard to such testing Timm (31) states that it should not be used, at this time, to qualify or disqualify a person from job activities on the basis of lifting performance ability. Rather, it provides a useful tool in a system of screening individuals for general lifting ability relative to a normal group.

Psychophysical Strength Testing

A third type of strength testing is referred to as psychophysical analysis. These are dynamic tests in which the worker is allowed to adjust the amount of load being lifted by adding or deleting weight. A tolerable load is determined by the worker, one that can be lifted with a frequency rate required by the particular task. This tolerable load is used to determine a safe upper limit for the worker. In a study

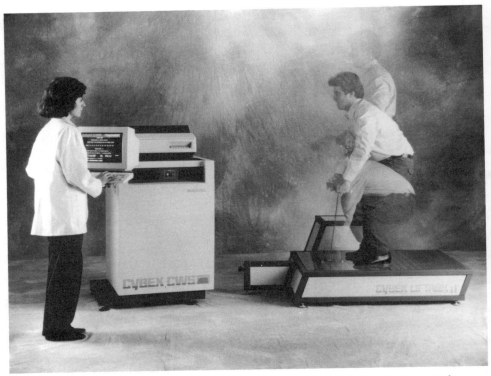

Figure 7.3. Cybex "Liftask." There are many objective testing devices that are used in the evaluation of back strength. (Photo courtesy of Cybex, a division of Lumex, Inc.)

by Griffin et al. (43) workers with a history of previous back pain chose lower acceptable loads than those without prior back problems. Chaffin (39) feels that this may be a most reliable and accurate method of assessing a workers performance. Troup et al. (44), however, in a 1-year study of 2891 men and women found only a 35 and 37% predictive value, respectively.

X-rays

X-rays of the lumbar spine have been used for many years and have probably been the most widely used pre-employment test. In my early years in practice (during the mid-1970s) I x-rayed the lumbar spines of many prospective railroad workers. One individual with a grade 2 spondylolisthesis was turned down for employment based solely on that single finding. Mandell et al. (6) claim that somewhere between

7.5 and 60 million dollars are still spent annually on pre-employment x-rays.

Unfortunately, the use of such procedures is difficult to support. The body of knowledge is such that the condition of the x-ray seems to have little correlation with the condition of the patient and the routine use of pre-employment x-rays, unless specifically indicated by the history and/or physical examination findings, is discouraged.

Psychosocial Factors

With all of the evidence indicating a strong link between the psychosocial risk factors and the development and severity of back pain it would seem prudent to use some type of evaluation in this area. Perhaps the use of instruments such as those listed here might be incorporated:

a. Minnesota Multiphasic Personality Inventory (MMPI)
b. Schedule of Recent Experience (SRE) (45)
c. Personal Concerns Inventory (PCI) (46)
d. Sickness Impact Profile (SIP) (47)
e. Quality of Well-being Scale (QWB) (48)

It should be apparent to the reader that, as it is with the treatment of back pain, no single test or screening procedure will provide all the necessary information to accurately predict the future industrial back injury. Rather, the problem must be viewed with the same multifactorial approach as with the etiology and management.

ERGONOMICS

Ergonomics is defined as the study of the relationship between a worker and his working environment. This field incorporates a broad knowledge of occupational biomechanics, engineering, kinesiology and physiology as well as a thorough understanding of the health and safety guidelines established by NIOSH. As such, it is beyond the scope of this text and is probably beyond the scope of most practicing chiropractors. While many chiropractors continue to make suggestions regarding safe lifting procedures and back safety measures, including minor modifications in the work station, major modifications should probably be left to those more qualified in this complex and ever-changing field. It is suggested that the chiropractor who is particularly interested in this area join forces with a trained ergonomist and work as a team. The prevention of back injury in the workplace is, after all, a team effort.

The Seated Workplace

One area that is relatively easy to approach in the area of ergonomics, and one that is often not considered as a primary factor in the development of back pain, is the seated workplace (Fig. 7.4). An increasing number of workers spend their work day, not engaged in any heavy labor, but seated at a desk, a workbench, or a computer terminal. Often the posture of this seated worker remains unchanged throughout the day and the potential for muscle fatigue and back strains is rather great. Added to this is the increase in psychological stress that often accompanies such jobs. Consequently, a review of some of the factors that influence muscle fatigue and productivity is included here.

When work is performed in the seated posture many factors influence the neck, shoulders, lower back, and lower limbs. The seated posture is dependent upon the design of the chair, the design of the workstation and tools to be used, the lighting, and the postural habits of the individual. The following factors have been identified as having a direct influence on muscle fatigue and intradiscal pressures (48):

a. Inclination of the backrest
b. The use of a lumbar support
c. The use of an armrest
d. Worktable height
e. Inclination of the seatrest

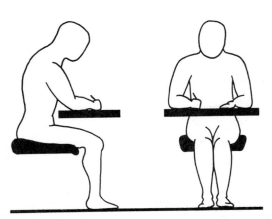

Figure 7.4. The seated worker is vulnerable to back injuries. (Adapted from Donkin SW. Sitting on the Job. Lincoln, NE: Parallel Integration, 1987.)

It has been my experience that the modification of the worksta-tion can make a substantial difference in the recovery of the injured patient and in the prevention of other stress-related problems such as cervical tension headaches, thoracic outlet syndromes, carpal tunnel syndromes, etc.

References

1. Brandt-Rauf PW, Brandt-Rauf SI. History of occupational medicine: relevance of Imhotep and Edwin Smith papyrus. Br J Ind Med 1987;44:68.
2. Horal J. The clinical appearance of low back pain disorders in the city of Gothenburg, Sweden. Acta Orthop Scand Suppl 1969;1(118):109.
3. Kelsey JL. An epidemiological survey of the relationship between occupation and acute herniated lumbar intervertebral disc. Int J Epidemiol 1975;4:197–205.
4. Snook SH, Campanelli RA, Ford RJ. A study of back injuries at Pratt and Whitney Aircraft. Hopkinton, MA: Liberty Mutual Insurance Company, Research Center, 1980.
5. Magora A. Investigation of the relation between low back pain and occupation: Age, sex, community, education and other factors. Ind Med Surg 1972 ;39:465–471.
6. Mandell P, Lipton MH, Bernstein J, Kucera GJ, Kaupner JA. Low Back Pain. Thorofare, NJ: Slack Inc. 1989:3.
7. Snook SH, Campanelli RA, Ford RJ. A study of three preventive approaches to low back injury. J Occup Med 1978;20:478.
8. Hult L. Cervical, dorsal and lumbar spine syndromes. Acta Orthop Scand Suppl 1954;17:102.
9. Kelsey JL, Hardy RL. Driving of motor vehicles as a risk factor for acute herniated lumbar intervertebral disc. Am J Epidemiol 1975;102:63–73.
10. Afacan AS. Sickness absence due to back lesions in coal miners. J Soc Occup Med 1982;32:26–31.
11. Undeutsch K. Back complaints and findings in transport workers performing physically heavy work. Scand J Work Environ Health 1982;8(suppl 1):92–96.
12. Venning PJ, Walter SD, Stitt LW. Personal and job-related factors as determi-nants of incidence of back injuries among nursing personnel. J Occup Med 1987;29(10):820–825.
13. Deyo RA, Tsui-Wu YJ. Descriptive epidemiology of low back pain and its related medical care in the United States. Spine 1987;3:268.
14. Kirkaldy-Willis WH. Managing low back pain. New York: Churchill-Livingstone, 1988:5.
15. Lewit K. Manipulative therapy in rehabilitation of the locomotor system. London: Butterworths, 1985:26.
16. Mierau DR, Cassidy JD, Hamin T, Milne RA. Sacroiliac joint dysfunction and low back pain in school aged children. J Manipulative Physiol Ther 1984;7(2):81–84.
17. Gyntelberg F. One year incidence of low back pain among male residents of Copenhagen aged 40–59. Dan Med Bull 1974;21:30–36.
18. Hrubec Z, Nashold BS. Epidemiology of lumbar disc lesions in the military in World War II. Am J Epidemiol 1975;102:366–376.
19. Manning DP. Slipping accidents causing low back pain in a gearbox factory. Spine 1981;6:70–72.

20. Brennan GP, Ruhling RO, Hood RS, Shultz BB, Johnson SC, Andrews BC. Physical characteristics of patients with herniated intervertebral lumbar discs. *Spine* 1987;12(7):699–702.
21. Heliovarra M. Body height, obesity, and risk of herniated lumbar intervertebral disc. *Spine* 1987;5:469–471.
22. Sprangfort EV. The lumbar disc herniation, a computer-aided analysis of 2504 operations. *Acta Orthop Scand Suppl* 1972;142.
23. Kelsey JL, Ostfeld AM. Demographic characteristics of persons with acute herniated lumbar intervertebral disc. *J Chronic Dis* 1975;28:37.
24. Chaffin DB, Park KS. A longitudinal study of low back pain as associated with occupation with lifting factors. *Am Ind Hgy Assoc J* 1973;34:513–525.
25. Steinberg GS. The epidemiology of low back pain. Stanton-Hicks M, Boas R, eds. New York: Raven Press, 1982;1–12.
26. Cady LD, Bischoff DP, O'Connell ER, Thomas PC, Allen JH. Strength and fitness and subsequent back injuries in firefighters. *J Occup Med* 1979;21:269–272.
27. Alston W, Carlson KE, Feldman DJ, Grimm Z, Gerontinos E. A quantitative study of muscle factors in the chronic low back syndrome. *J Am Geriat Soc* 1966;14:1041–1047.
28. Biering-Sorensen F. A one-year prospective study of low back trouble in a general population. *Dan Med Bull* 1984;31(5):362–375.
29. Suzuki N, Endo S. A quantitative study of trunk muscle strength and fatigability in the low back pain syndrome. *Spine* 1983;1:69–74.
30. Nachemson A, Lindh M. Measurement of abdominal and back muscle strength with and without low back pain. *Scand J Rehabil Med* 1969;1:60–65.
31. Timm KE. Isokinetic lifting simulation: a normative data study. *J Orthop Sports Ther* Nov. 1988;156–166.
32. Frymoyer JW, Pope MH, Costanza MC, et al. Epidemiologic studies of low back pain. *Spine* 1980;5:419.
33. Nachemson AL, Elfstrom G. Intravital dynamic pressure measurements in lumbar discs. *Scand J Rehabil Med Suppl* 1970;1.
34. Daniell HW. Osteoporosis of the slender smoker. *Arch Intern Med* 1976;136:298.
35. Frymoyer JW, Pope MH, Clements FH, et al. Risk factors in low back pain: an epidemiological survey. *J Bone Joint Surg* 1983;65A:213.
36. Vallfors B. Acute, sub-acute and chronic low back pain, clinical symptoms, absenteeism and working environment. *Scand J Rehabil Med* 1985;11:1–98.
37. Deyo RA, Tsui-Wu YJ. Functional disability due to back pain; a population based study indicating the importance of socioeconomic factors. *Arthritis Rheum* 1987;30:1247.
38. Lloyd DCEF, Troup JDG. Recurrent back pain and its prediction. *J Soc Occup Med* 1983;33:66–74.
39. Chaffin DB, Andersson G. *Occupational biomechanics.* New York: John Wiley & Sons, 1984:89–109.
40. Chaffin DB, Herin GD, Keyserling WM. Pre-employment strength-testing; an updated position. *J Occup Med* 1978;20(6):403–408.
41. Keyserling WM, Herrin GD, Chaffin DB, et al. Establishing an industrial strength testing program. *Am Ind Hyg Assoc J* Oct. 1980;730–736.
42. Keyserling WM, Herrin GD, Chaffin DB, et al. Isometric strength testing as a means of controlling medical accidents on strenuous jobs. *J Occup Med* 1980;22(5):332–336.

43. Griffin AB, Troup JDG, Lloyd DCEF. Tests of lifting and handling capacity: their repeatability and relationship to back symptoms. *Ergonomics* 1984;27:305–320.

44. Troup JDG, Foreman TK, Baxter CE, Brown D. The perception of back pain and the role of psycholphysical tests of lifting capacity. Spine 1987;12(7):645–657.

45. Meyers JE. Overview by industry of lumbar spine pain problems. In: *AAOS: Symposium on the Lumbar Spine.* Brown FW, ed. St. Louis: C.V. Mosby, 1981:193–202.

46. Mulry R. A functional psychological approach to low back pain. In: *AAOS: Symposium on the Lumbar Spine.* Brown FW, ed. St. Louis: C.V. Mosby, 1981:117–125.

47. McDowell I, Newell C. *Measuring health, a guide to rating scales and questionnaires.* New York: Oxford University Press, 1987:290–295.

48. Chaffin DB, Andersson G. *Occupational biomechanics.* New York: John Wiley & Sons, 1984:289–323.

8

Factors That Influence Compliance

The major thrust of this text has been the identification and elimination of the causes of back pain, especially recurring back pain. As described, this incorporates many different components including: (a) worker selection techniques, (b) redesigning the workplace, (c) an increase in the use of active patient participation in treatment programs through exercise programs, etc., and (d) patient education programs. It is hoped that the combination of approaches discussed will gradually reduce the impact of this expensive and disabling problem.

As an educator, my primary interest for the past number of years has been in improving the patient's understanding of their back and in promoting the Back School in the chiropractic profession. In any discussion of the Back School as a means of patient education, two questions must be considered: 1) does the patient actually understand what is expected of him/her?; and 2) does the patient actually comply with the instructions given? In this chapter we will discuss the various factors that influence patient compliance, the correlation between compliance and the successful achievement of treatment goals, and methods of determining patient compliance.

The primary purpose of the Back School, as part of a comprehensive approach to the problem of back pain, is to change the behavior of the back pain patient. The patient must learn a variety of new ways of dealing with pain, new ways of accomplishing common tasks, and perhaps even a new occupation. The patient may even be asked to stop doing certain activities that s/he enjoys. In order to accomplish this the patient must be willing to take the time necessary to learn such new activities. In addition, the patient must actually make the changes required. All this requires a great deal of effort and attention by the individual.

Whether or not the patient actually follows through with the treatment prescribed, does the exercises as instructed, makes the changes in daily activities, stops harmful activities, etc. is a problem in and of itself. The cooperation of the patient with the recommendations of the physician is referred to as "patient compliance," a most complex and, from the clinicians point of view, frustrating topic. To further frustrate the clinician, the fact that the patient does or does not comply with the proposed regimen is no guarantee of the outcome. The compliant patient is not guaranteed success, nor is the noncompliant patient guaranteed failure.

Of the many unanswered questions in the area of Back School programs is the compliance of the patient with the recommendations made. Does the patient actually make the necessary lifestyle changes? If so, what triggers them to act in a productive way? If not, what motivates, or fails to motivate, them to behave in a manner that is very likely counterproductive to their own well-being? Linton and Kanwendo (1) state that there are almost no data available concerning whether patients do comply with the instructions they receive in low back schools. In fact, they claim most of the data indicates that patients do not significantly alter their behavior (1). Lankhorst (2) found that only 12 of 20 patients attending a particular back school actually used the information they were provided.

A second question is, "Did the patient actually understand what s/he was taught?" It is obvious that in order for a patient to comply with instructions, they must first understand them. To those of us involved in education, whether in the classroom or in the clinic, the ability of the individual student to grasp information is an ongoing concern. The simple fact that a student has been given facts does not mean they will understand or remember them. A teacher must constantly evaluate whether the information provided was meaningful, whether it was organized in such a way that makes learning easy, whether the methods used in transferring the information to the student were effective, and whether the instructor was able to motivate the student to continue learning once the class was over. Some studies such as that of Hultman et al. (3) indicate that individual participants are more informed after attending low back school. On the other hand, Dehlin et al. (4) saw no change in lifting techniques despite efforts at education.

While it is not clear whether or not the majority of individuals attending a back school program actually modify their behavior, it is clear that the attitudes of the participants are positively affected (5). This in itself will influence compliance.

COMPLIANCE

Health care education is undertaken with the goal of changing the behavior of individuals. An understanding of the nature of things that influence this behavior is essential to anyone interested in the Back School. Consequently, it is important that we consider the factors that influence patient compliance and attempt to understand its complexities.

Compliance may be described in a variety of ways. In the context of health education, compliance is associated with the extent to which an individual carries out a prescribed regimen. To this end it nearly always involves a change in the behavior of the individual. This may include some modification in activity such as using new lifting techniques or asking for help when confronted with a particularly heavy object. It may include modifying the chair of the office worker to make the workstation more comfortable or perhaps even purchasing a more ergonomically designed chair. It may involve adding a new activity such as an exercise program or taking vitamin supplements. It may simply be the addition of a weekly trip to the Back School or to the chiropractor. In some cases it may involve deleting some harmful activity from the individuals lifestyle, perhaps giving up smoking or alcohol or losing weight.

Some equate compliance with the achievement of a treatment goal. In other words, many assume that if a patient complies s/he will respond. If s/he does not comply, s/he will not respond. This is not, unfortunately, an accurate way of measuring patient compliance. Some patients follow the doctors instructions to the letter and yet fail to respond. Others seem to ignore all advice and recover, it seems, in spite of themselves. When investigating the relationship between the treatment goals and compliance two factors must be considered: 1) the validity of the goal, and 2) the efficacy of the regimen.

First, let's consider the validity of the goal. Each of us involved in aspects of patient care establish goals, whether verbalized to the patient or not. The success of our treatment is determined based on whether or not we attain these goals. A most important step in the administering of care is the establishment of reasonable, attainable goals. It would not be reasonable to expect a patient in the terminal stages of cancer to reach a pain-free state for an extended period of time. Neither would it be reasonable to expect a patient with a 20-year history of back pain who has been diagnosed as having a "failed surgical back syndrome" to reach a completely pain-free condition. It would certainly be reasonable, however, to strive for a reduction in the degree and intensity of pain in either patient.

One patient seen by this author was a 63-year-old engineer. He described a lengthy history of back problems including several surgeries. He complained of a chronic, unrelenting back pain but his primary concern was a claudicant pain in the calves upon walking. He was unable to walk even a few blocks without extreme pain. Upon radiographic examination it was evident that he had advanced central stenosis, a condition that was not likely to go away. Treatment goals were established and agreed upon between the patient and myself. These goals were able to guide both the treatment that he received and the level of activity that he engaged in. It would have been most unreasonable to expect this patient to walk several miles each day. This, however, was his ultimate goal. Walking had always been an activity that he enjoyed and was his primary form of relaxation. Consequently, we first set a goal of walking two blocks without pain in his legs. This took nearly 1 month to attain but he was elated when we finally accomplished this. Upon accomplishing this first goal we doubled the distance for the next step, 4 blocks without pain. Again this took a considerable amount of time but was something that we both agreed was worth working toward. With the achievement of each progressive improvement we established new goals. Much like the morbidly obese dieter who gauges success in 10-pound increments, it was important to establish goals that he could reach. Without constant positive reinforcement many people stop trying and give up.

The second component that we must consider in relating the compliance with the achievement of a treatment goal is the efficacy of the regimen. If the treatment regimen or self-care activities prescribed are ineffective at dealing with the problem at hand, then success is unlikely. For example, disc surgery is unlikely to provide much relief to a patient who suffers from a piriformis syndrome due to myofascial trigger points. Likewise, a program of stretching exercises would not be as likely to help a ballet dancer or gymnast who is already extremely flexible. It is important to realize that each treatment regimen, each exercise protocol, each modification in ADL is going to probably help some patients. No treatment regimen, exercise protocol, etc. is going to help all patients. It is imperative that the methods used, whether they be passive or active, be tailored to the individual. It is also imperative that the progress of the individual be monitored continually and changes in the approach made as indicated by the success or failure of the plan.

Rather than an absolute, that is, patients comply completely or not at all, it is more realistic to describe compliance as a process. The ultimate result of this process is ideally, but not totally, a positive change in the health behavior of the individual. With this view, compliance may be seen not as a goal in and of itself but as a process that may lead to the achievement of a goal.

This process of compliance involves three major elements: 1) cognition, 2) attitude, and 3) behavior (6).

Cognition

Before an individual is able to comply with a regimen, s/he must first know and understand what it is s/he is being asked to do and how and when it is to be done. Some people also need to know why the particular treatment plan or exercises have been prescribed and the consequences of not following through. It has been stated that if a patient does not know what to do, s/he cannot comply. Unfortunately, just because a patient does know what is expected of them does not mean that s/he will comply.

Attitude

Before an individual can accomplish anything, be it changing work habits, performing exercises, losing weight, etc. s/he must be willing to fulfill the various aspects of the plan. Most overweight people know how to lose weight, expend more calories than you take in. The problem with many would-be dieters is they do not have the desire to actually do that. And so it is with the back-injured patient. S/he must be willing to take time to exercise, to take a walk after the evening meal instead of having dessert, or to change the way s/he lifts at work, etc. The patient who is in the midst of a medico-legal battle over compensation for an injury at work may not be as willing to assist him/herself until the legal issues are settled.

Behavior

Finally, even if the individual knows what is expected of him/her, and is willing to comply, necessary changes must actually be made. In other words, *they* must actually change. They must lift using safer lifting techniques. They must actually perform the exercises prescribed for them on a regular basis. They must push themselves away from the table. It is frustrating for the doctor to hear a patient who presents in pain state, "I know better than to do that, but I did it anyway." One patient I saw who presented with an acute episode of low back pain hurt his back while lifting a riding lawn mower out of the back of his pickup truck, unassisted. Since this was not the first time that he had hurt his back doing the same thing he was not the least bit surprised. He told me, "I knew I should get help but I was in a hurry."

In summary, compliance is a complex concept that is closely related to patient care. It cannot, however, be directly related to the achievement of a treatment goal. Compliance, even in the most well-intentioned and informed patient tends to vacillate. The fact that the patient does comply one day does not guarantee that s/he will comply the next. Many factors enter into the ultimate behavior of the patient with regard to passive treatment and self-care. These factors will be discussed in the following sections.

NONCOMPLIANCE

Noncompliance is the other end of the spectrum and absorbs a great deal of time and energy of the health care industry. Estimates of noncompliance range from 20% to as high as 60%. Some cite even higher rates, especially in those who are free of symptoms. A reasonable estimate is 50%. To put this in perspective, consider the female patient who presents to the medical doctor with a urinary tract infection and is given a 10-day supply of antibiotics. Within a few days the symptoms begin to improve and by the fifth day she is symptom-free. How frequently does the woman continue to take the medication for the entire 10 days? How much more frequently does she stop the medication once the symptoms are gone and keep the medicine in the cabinet until the next occurrence? Whether or not the additional medication would have had any significant impact on her condition is not the issue. The fact is, this situation serves to illustrate noncompliance.

The consequences of noncompliance are difficult to gauge and vary considerably. Noncompliance may:

1. Compromise the patient's health status. Failure to stop smoking and lower cholesterol and blood pressure levels in the patient recovering from a heart attack may have fatal consequences.
2. May delay or even prevent recovery from a particular condition. The patient who discontinues care at the first sign of symptom relief may continue to worsen.
3. May increase the number and cost of additional procedures. The patient recovering from an open fracture who discontinues antiobiotic therapy too soon may suffer from osteomyelitis that requires surgical intervention.

Each of us, as health care providers and educators find our job more difficult in the face of noncompliance. When faced with the noncompliant patient we must attempt to determine the reason. When faced with the unresponsive patient we must assess whether the problem results from noncompliance, from an ineffective method or approach to the patient, from an incorrect diagnosis, or a combination of these.

COMPLIANCE VERSUS NONCOMPLIANCE

The reasons that motivate a patient to follow, or not to follow, a prescribed course of treatment are not consistent from one patient to the next. Some patients do not follow through because they simply did not understand what it was they were to do. Some understood initially but forgot. Others do not comply for a variety of reasons, both conscious and unconscious. Consider the patient who was injured at work on an assembly line. He dislikes his job and his supervisors and feels that the company is "out to get him." After being off work for several weeks, during which time he has been inactive, he is told by the company doctor that he must return to work or risk losing his job. He returns grudgingly and reinjures his weakened back. This time, at the suggestion of a friend who had received a large settlement for a similar injury and who had been granted early retirement, he enlists the advice of an attorney who tells him of the financial "potential" of his case. At this point, compliance with a regimen that is designed to make him pain-free and return him to work (at a job he dislikes) is almost counterproductive in his eyes.

Compliance and noncompliance are really two ends of a single continuum. No patient is fixed at any one point for any length of time. Rather, they move from one point to another as their situations and their conditions change.

FACTORS INFLUENCING COMPLIANCE

Some of the factors that determine compliance or noncompliance are listed here.

Knowledge

As stated before, if a patient does not know or understand what is expected of them, s/he cannot comply. Patient education, in itself, is not the solution, however. Simply because the patient understands does not mean that s/he will comply. This relationship between compliance and knowledge is best summarized by the statement, "While knowledge does not presume compliance, it must be present for compliance to occur."

The Relationship with the Provider

This may be one of the most important aspects that determines patient cooperation with a treatment program. There are several factors that influence this component. Some exert a negative influence, others a positive one.

The negative factors are:

a. Incongruent expectations between the patient and the provider. The patient in acute pain who is unable to walk, sit, or get out of bed is not interested in efforts to rehabilitate his/her spine or to prevent reinjury. His/her only interest at the moment is relief of pain. Once this is accomplished, other things may be considered. The doctor who fails to recognize this encounters a patient who may become agitated and seek help elsewhere.
b. Dissatisfaction with the relationship between the patient and the provider. The manner in which the patient perceives the provider may have a drastic effect on compliance. If, for some reason, the patient is unhappy with the encounter, perhaps s/he may have been treated too abruptly by a staff member who appeared more interested in the insurance reimbursement than in the care of the patient, compliance is negatively affected.

On the positive side, it has been observed that adherence is greater when:

a. The patient's expectations have been met.
b. The provider asks about and respects all of the patient's concerns.
c. The patient and provider agree on specifics of the regimen.
d. The patient perceives the doctor as listening to his/her concerns, explaining the condition in easily understood terms, and considering the patient's feelings and concerns when planning treatment.

Social Support

It is most likely that the support of family and friends is necessary for compliance on any long-term basis. Consider the patient who learns an exercise regimen at a Back School, only to be told by a hostile spouse that there is really nothing wrong with them in the first place. It is alarming how frequently a well-meaning dieter is sabotaged by an unsupportive spouse. Whenever a patient begins a therapeutic regimen there is a simultaneous effect on the circle of family and friends. The degree to which the relationship between the patient and the individuals in this circle is disrupted by the prescribed regimen will often influence the patient's willingness to comply. Our attempts to educate patients via the Back School are enhanced whenever the family and friends can be included in the process. For this reason, it may be advisable to hold special Back School training sessions for the family and friends of patients.

Health Belief Model

This is an example of a value-expectancy model. Decisions about whether or not to comply with a program depend on: 1) the value the patient has placed on the outcome, and 2) the patient's estimate of the likelihood of success if they do comply. These decisions are influenced by:

a. The patient's perception of their own susceptibility to a disease or their belief in the accuracy of the diagnosis.
b. The belief that the disease or the condition will actually have consequences on the patient's life.
c. The belief that the proposed course of action will reduce the

susceptibility to the condition or be effective in controlling the current problem.

d. Any barriers to the proposed course of action must be surmountable. These barriers may be real or perceived.

e. The existence of some type of triggering mechanism or cue to action. The patient in acute pain is usually willing to comply with any suggestion to provide help. Once the pain is gone, however, patient compliance becomes much more fragile. How frequently have we seen a patient dedicate themselves to an exercise regimen or a treatment program for a period of several months, only to disappear once the symptoms are gone. Months later, the patient returns, once again in pain.

The Patient's Values

The values that the individual holds about their health and related issues greatly affect their willingness to seek care and to follow the recommendations provided. Each patient faces a wide array of competing demands for his/her time, money, energy, and attention and health care is only one of these. The patient who is asked to give up an activity, such as a sport that s/he places a high value on is less likely to comply than the patient who is asked to give up an activity that s/he does not enjoy. Compliance, from the patient's point of view, is really a series of tradeoffs in which the patient gives up or takes on certain behaviors in return for some promised benefit.

The Treatment Plan

One of the most important factors influencing compliance is the treatment plan itself. In other words, what exactly is the patient being asked to do? Some cite this as one of the most important of all potential impediments or enhancers of compliance.

SUMMARY

Throughout this text I have attempted to discuss the complex nature of the back pain problem. Several different aspects involving treatment as well as education have been presented in an effort to modify the intensity of the problem and reduce the frequency of recurrence. All of this, however, falls apart in the face of the noncompliant patient. All of the good intentions in the world do no good unless some action is taken.

One of the principal messages of this text is that, ultimately it is the patient who is responsible for his/her back. It is not the responsibility of the doctor, the employer, the insurance company, or anyone else. The patient *must* accept the final responsibility. Only then can we hope to solve this costly and frustrating problem.

Over the years I have had the opportunity to view the back pain problem from a number of different perspectives. As a clinician I was intimately involved in the complex process of diagnosing and treating patients suffering from back pain of varying degree. As a chiropractor, I felt that if only the rest of the unresolved back problems which appeared in the records of other doctors could have the benefit of my skill and expertise this would be much less of a problem. This somewhat egotistical viewpoint has been gradually tempered over the years by the patients who, for whatever reason, did not respond to my care.

As an educator, I have been interested in the process involved in teaching the back pain patient to alter the course of their condition. It is my firm belief that this particular component holds much more promise than we are currently able to substantiate in the literature. Our methods of education need to improve, however. It is unrealistic to compare the results of different Back Schools when the curriculum, the teaching methods, the training of the instructors and the patient population remains so varied. Perhaps part of the solution to this lies in the colleges doing a better job of preparing the modern chiropractor to fulfill his/her role as a patient educator.

As a patient, I have directly benefited from activities directed at preventing future recurrences of a chronic back problem. My own problem is in my hands. Any future back problems that I have, barring any unforseen major injuries, are my own doing. Even in the event of a major injury, my reaction to such is in my hands.

Finally, I would like to relate a story that, to me, graphically illustrates my belief. I have a very close friend who, approximately 1 year ago, fell and injured his back. The fall occurred on the job shortly before Christmas. The fall was witnessed by several co-workers and reported to his supervisor. The following day my friend (for convenience I will call him Frank) left on a week-long vacation during which he drove several thousand miles to visit relatives. I am sure that this aggravated his condition and, by the time he returned home, he was in a sad state.

At his request, I referred him to a local chiropractor whom I knew. He was examined and treated for a herniated intervertebral disc for the next several months. The treatment produced some positive symptomatic response but no real change in the condition, so Frank voluntarily discontinued care. The total bill for services rendered, at this point, was probably less than one thousand dollars.

For the next few months my friend did nothing. His condition remained about the same, neither improving nor worsening. A few months later he was contacted by the insurance provider who inquired as to his current status. When told that he still had some pain the provider requested an "independent medical examination" (IME). The examiner, to my surprise, found Frank to be in good health and suggested he was "permanent and stationary" and could expect no further progress and needed no further treatment. In my opinion, this was a turning point in this situation. Frank was perturbed by the IME and expressed his dissatisfaction to the insurance carrier. Some 2 months later, at Frank's request, a second IME was performed by the same examiner. Needless to say, the examiner agreed with his original examination and found my friend to have no problems.

At this point, Frank became somewhat agitated by the process. He expressed to me that his back hurt. He did not seem to want any remuneration for his injury. He simply wanted to not hurt any longer. At Frank's request, the examiner ordered a magnetic resonance imaging (MRI) of his lumbar spine. However, the examiner cautioned Frank that there was a significant chance that the MRI would be positive for a disc bulge at the level indicated. This was not, he was told, of any real significance as a large percentage of normal people had a positive MRI or computerized tomography (CT).

A few days later, the examiner was contacted by the radiology group that interpreted the MRI. Frank had a 6-mm bulge of the L4-5 disc. Confirmation, in Frank's mind of the severity of his injury. Remember that he had mild to moderate residual pain prior to the first IME. Now he had a "serious" problem. The story becomes particularly interesting at this point. The examiner who did the first two IMEs realized that this was a patient with a structural problem. To the examiner this meant "disability." To my friend, this was confirmation that his pain was real. I'm not sure whether he was more concerned by the finding or pleased that he really did have a reason for his pain.

My friend was immediately referred to a neurosurgeon who recommended surgery as the only alternative (to the man with a hammer in his hand, everything looks like a nail). At my request, Frank saw a neurologist who gave him alternatives to surgery (I had also given him alternatives but I think Frank only wanted my sympathy, not my advice).

The neurologist basically told Frank that his condition was in his hands. He could have surgery and maybe he would be better off. Maybe not. Or he could exercise, change his activities, and resolve the problem. Frank seemed, at this point, pleased that he did not have to have surgery. He telephoned me for my advice regarding what exercises he could do and was excited. Unfortunately, to this day, Frank has not done any of the things that I suggested.

In the meantime, the examiner who did the initial IME telephoned Frank and told him that he should consult an attorney because he was entitled to some type of compensation for this injury. (Appreciate that this is the same individual who originally told Frank that there was nothing really wrong with him. Now, however, he had structural evidence of abnormality.) I think, regardless of Frank's intentions, morals, or situation, until he resolves the financial aspects of this case, he simply will not get better. Once this is taken care of, Frank may or may not improve. It's up to him.

I remain on the sidelines frustrated beyond belief. This has all occurred to my friend while I am writing this book on the very subject of chronic back pain. While I am sensitive to Frank's plight I have no sympathy. I am more convinced of the primary premise of this text: the ultimate responsibility for the resolution of back pain lies with the patient. If there is one single message that I would like the reader to take to heart, that's it!

References

1. Linton SJ, Kamwendo K. Low back schools: A critical review. *Phys Ther* 1987;67(9):1375–1383.
2. Lankhorst GJ, Van de Stadt RJ, Vogelaar TW, et al. The effect of the Swedish back school in chronic idiopathic low back pain—A prospective controlled study. *Scand J Rehab Med* 1983;15:141.
3. Hultman G, Nordin M, Ortengren R. The influence of a preventive educational programme on trunk flexion in janitors. *Appl Ergonomics* 1984;15:127–133.
4. Dehlin O, Hedenrud B, Horal J. Back symptoms in nursing aids in a geriatric hospital. *Scand J Rehab Med* 1976;8:47.
5. Hall H, Iceton JA. Back school: An overview with specific reference to the Canadian back education units. *Clin Orthop* 1983;179:10–17.
6. Meichenbaum D, Turk DC. *Facilitating Treatment Adherence*. New York: Plenum Press, 1987, pp. 41–64.

Index

Page numbers in *italics* denote figures.

153